MW00938580

HYPE

"Gregory Boytos IS pizza." J. Patrick Rigney, Hollywood Screenwriter

"Just eyes. Just frames. Just a hidden smile of comfort in your confidence that eating what you want will set you free." – Ben Goldsmith, Comedian

"Greg Boytos is hardcore. He makes jokes. He eats pizza. He runs. One time he ran so hard he almost died... Heed his humorous advice." – Stephanie Asher, Attorney

"15 Years ago, Greg lost my copy of The Big Lebowski. He was young and relatively foolish. Now, he's older and I look to him as a pioneer in pizza-based diets." – Jason Maslanka, Holder of Misguided Grudge

"I do remember thinking 'hmmm... why would anyone want to eat so much pizza?' But then remembering how novel, unique, and memorable that time was, congrats on making it into a worthy cause." – Frances Boytos, My Mom

"Wait. Do you have a book out?" – Dexter Thomas Jr., Real Actual Journalist

Gregory Boytos

THE GREAT PIZZA EXPERIMENT

How I ate nothing but pizza for 45 days and lost weight, and other stories

Gregory Boytos

Gregory Boytos

Cover designed by Scott Thiede swthiede@icloud.com

Gregory Boytos

Instagram: @thepizzathlete
www.gregoryboytos.com

Printed in the United States of America

First Printing: September 2018

ISBN: 9781723823701

This book is for my wife, Robin Boytos, who let me eat nothing but pizza for 45 days for almost no reason at all. This book is for my parents Frances and Andrew Boytos who let me eat mostly pizza for the first eighteen years of my life.
This book is also for pizza.

MENU

1. "GENESIS."

"Do you like podcasts?" My creative director was making polite conversation as we walked back from the kitchen with our morning cups of coffee. It was intended as just a bit of banter to make the walk less quiet, but I have never been a fan of small talk or filler or holding back on sharing my opinion. Lest I died too young I have been living in a manner to leave no doubt on any stance where I have one.

"No. There are too many of them, they're too long, they rarely are interesting, and I'd rather do almost anything else than sit still and listen to people talk and not be able to chime in." I wasn't lying, but the way he exhaled revealed that I was living up to my office nickname, "The Speed Bump," because no conversation ever passed over me without some difficulty.

"Some of them can be entertaining; downright thought provoking." He's English. He talks with semicolons. "For example. This morning, they were discussing if you had to choose one food and eat only that one food for the rest of your life, would you choose pizza or sandwiches?"

This was not interesting or entertaining. There was only one clear answer. I'm sure I pulled an awful face and waved my hand in dismissal. "Stupid. Pizza."

"I don't know, if you think about sandwiches— "

"But pizza is pizza."

"Hamburgers, pita bread, bagels, hot dogs, ice cream sandwiches, Diddy Reese— "

"Fuck all of them. Pizza."

He didn't get it. He started to list off more sandwiches and I pulled in a coworker to vote. That dumb dumb said sandwiches. The next person walking past and trying to mind their own business voted sandwiches as well and that's when I had to walk away. Surrounded by idiots was never a good position but there I was, and my coffee was getting cold.

I put the question out social media and was shocked to see so many people whom I formerly respected air out their ignorance on the world wide web. Had they never had pizza? Were their parents killed by pizza and now they were holding a grudge? What kind of tuna melt were they eating to make pizza sound so terrible? What happened to them to make them all have the wrong thought?

Pizza is objectively not only preferable to sandwiches, but also it is the best single food that exists. It has all the food groups in the right ratios for consumption. It is beyond delicious. Its utility does not diminish. Pizza may in fact be perfect.

I know there are a lot of problems with the standard American diet. It may not work for everyone, but it is the most reasonable, affordable and healthful diet that will work the best for the most people. It's the food pyramid. We all know what it looks like: the base is grains, then fruits and vegetables, dairy, protein and then on top sweets.

Everyone could agree the first thing you would want to eliminate from your diet to improve it would be sweets, right? Pizza does that. Have you ever had chocolate on a pizza? I'm not talking about dessert pizza, that's a different, also amazing thing. I'm talking about pizza pizza. With sauce. Yeah. You leave that sweets stuff off. Except graham crackers. If you ever crumble those bad boys onto a slice of cheese pizza you will not be sorry. Graham crackers aside, normal pizza is decidedly free from sweets and excessive sugar.

I'm not going to spell out how perfectly balanced pizza is for you. If you can't plainly see the right ratios of grain in the crust, vegetables in the sauce – and sparingly as toppings to maintain good flavor, fruit and protein atop a light dusting of cheese, then I don't know how you've survived long enough to learn how to read. When God designed the food pyramid, She was eating pizza. But not every food is judged solely on nutrition.

Pop quiz. You can eat anything you want right now. Yeah, your brain went to that pizza from the place across town. The one your friend used to live near but then he moved in with his girlfriend and they don't really hang out all that often and when they do it's just drinks or dinner parties and wine, and even if they did hang they don't live near that place anymore so you'd have to go alone, so you never go anymore but you wish you did. Instead you sigh, peel yourself off the couch and eat whatever boring shit you have already in your fridge. Yeah. A sandwich. Sounds like a great food.

Pop quiz again. You have five bucks and you're starving. Like. You had to skip breakfast for a blood test and then you got a call while you were walking to your car and they need you at work right away! But after you put out the fires it's lunch time, but also payday isn't until tomorrow hence the five dollars, what do you do? Yeah. Two slices and a soda. Don't lie to me. don't lie to yourself.

Pop quiz again number 2! Do you know anyone who actually has celiac? When they go to get burgers with you do they eat the bun? No. they don't. Food allergies are serious, and you do not mess with them. But here's the pop quiz: your friend Simon is lactose intolerant. How do you know this? Every time that dude eats pizza he takes a deep sigh first, and you always ask, "What's up, man?"

"I'm lactose. This is gonna hurt," he always says. But does he avoid it? No. because pizza has that pull.

My nephew once ate so much pizza that he puked. Now, don't get me wrong, I loved the kid the day he dropped, but I didn't respect him until that day. For the rest of our lives, every time that kid eats pizza we will warn him not to eat too much otherwise he will. My nephew is alive.

This may seem like it flies in the face of a basic tenet of Economics: the law of diminishing marginal utility. It does. Pizza is special enough where its utility remains constant until the law of increasing marginal guilt makes us stop eating pizza. You've never had a second slice and thought to yourself, "self, that second slice was not as good as the first," because that never happens to normal people unless the first one had graham crackers and then you ran out of graham crackers, or you're a strange person with a questionable palate. Ever known anyone to have a second sandwich? Probably not.

Pop quiz: what food has balanced nutrition, is above the law of the free market to which we're all bound, tastes so good it makes people ignore their allergies causing them great pain and discomfort? This question is rhetorical, but the answer is also pizza. Pizza is all of those things. With the truth being thusly illuminated, and previously being so clear to me I could not fathom a universe where rational people, by whom I believed I was surrounded could think any differently, but they did.

I distilled it to three distinct camps: the first were those who felt restricted by pizza, the second were those who felt pizza was unhealthy, the third were trolls just arguing to argue.

Those who advocated for sandwiches from a variety perspective were wrong. Think about your last ten meals, how many were repeats? By repeat I mean food genre. There's standard meal with protein and carb and maybe a vegetable, soups, salads, sandwiches, noodle stuff and then probably a thousand other one-offs that are clever exceptions – which we'll use to briefly dismiss trolls. Trolls are never wrong, they just exploit oversights for simplicity's sake, so they can win petty arguments. But in all likelihood when you boil meals down to their basic genre, you likely repeat a bunch and it is for this reason that I dismiss the lack of variety argument against pizza. Our food variety is overestimated for sure, and this doesn't even delve into the incredibly beautiful diversity of pizza possibilities.

Crusts are quite basic, but for every sandwich bread option there is a corresponding pizza crust option because a pizza crust is bread. Though have you ever asked your sandwich artist or the PHD in sociology at your local independent coffee roaster / café for thick bread on your pastrami on rye? They'd probably look at you like you were crazy. That's not a thing! A bread slice only is one thickness: however it's already cut. Hell, even if they cut it from the rustic loaf right in front of you, you're never even given the option of thickness, and if you ask they'll roll their eyes at you and tweet about that unhinged customer who had a special request for bread thickness on their sandwich and only put a dollar into their tip jar on an eight dollar order. Their anonymous twitter account only has a couple hundred followers but one of them works at BuzzFeed and thinks that's an interesting anecdote, so they include it in their next "what all sandwich artists want you to STOP doing," listicle. You know who won't tweet about you? A pizza maker who gives you the crust option up front. To be sure: thick crust sourdough pizza is bucket-list worthy.

Sauce is similarly limited but any aioli you can get on a sandwich you can get as a sauce on a pizza. I don't think this is necessarily a point for pizza or for sandwiches, but I'll take this opportunity to talk about myself. I used to eat ham sandwiches that were just ham cheese and bread. People at sandwich shops would never get it on the first try. No mayo? No mustard? No oil? No salt and pepper? Just ham cheese and bread? Once the girls at the sub shop across the street from my university wrote "this sandwich is boring!" on the wax paper, and when it was ready said "Greg's boring sandwich is ready," which is basically a hate crime. However boring that sandwich was, I survived the shame and now I enjoy a full complement of liquids on my sandwiches. But has a pizza place ever busted my chops when I ordered a plain cheese pizza? Hell no!

Cheese is a pretty basic thing just like the sauce, though unless you want to wait extra-long for your sandwich, the cheese probably won't be melted when you get it. That's fine.

Maybe you don't like melted cheese or hot sandwiches. You know what's great, though? If you said "cold pizza" you'd be right. That is delicious. It isn't hot or melty either and it's better than a normal sandwich because you probably are still high on life from having pizza for dinner the night before and the only thing better than having pizza for dinner is going to bed with a bellyful of pizza and knowing that you get to eat more for breakfast.

I originally wrote the end of that last paragraph as, "the only thing better than being high is getting high again," instead of all that pizza stuff but it just sounded super pathetic. The metaphor faded into its own tenuous premise and it was just me talking about drugs in a pizza story. This isn't about drugs, this is about pizza. But just so we all are on the same page, you know what's a pants-shittingly good meal to eat when you're too high to change the channel even though it's on the Spanish channel because they're the only people in LA who have the dodger game because the English feed is on that cable channel that nobody can get but the game ended two hours ago but also you're too high to find the remote and how do you change the channel on the cable box there's no buttons? Pizza.

Also, anything you can get in a sandwich you can get on a pizza. Except ice cream. A pizookie isn't a pizza, it's just a big cookie. We will discuss it later, but it's a horrendous fact that needs to be stated but it has no glory to it. Dessert pizza is severely lacking in ice cream and cookies. This is the point of most paragraphs where there is a clever pirouette that spins pizza out on top, but I really like pizookies and they're not pizza. But they're not sandwiches either so now we're just scorching the earth.

Those who thought pizza was unhealthy were wrong. Pizza is nutritionally perfectly balanced. I'm sure they were confusing, "pizza," with, "too much pizza," which is definitely unhealthy! Too much pizza is unhealthy. Too much sandwich is also unhealthy! Too much anything is by definition too much, and less preferable than the optimal amount.

The truth is, a great number of the people who chose sandwiches were only doing so to avoid being unhealthy. They would say things like "I wish I could eat nothing but pizza, but it'd kill me!" That not only exposes the common misconception of the healthiness of pizza, but casts doubt on anyone's decision from team sandwich because the question was never "what is better for you?" but, "what would you rather have?" And if health was not an issue, more people would rather have pizza!

In any case, sandwich was a winner, but I had my doubts as to the veracity of that vote, so I did what everyone who loses an internet contest does: pretended it never happened. It was hard at first. Working with people who would choose sandwich over slice was especially challenging. If I was ever disagreed with I felt that I had a duty to defend my position. If they were wrong about pizza they surely were wrong about this work thing, what the fuck did they know about anything?!

Later, the same creative director and I were meeting with our boss when he dragged up the past. I felt reinvigorated. My boss was from New Jersey. That's where pizza was from! Surely, he'd be on my side and shut this Englishman up! But no. the traitor leaned back in his chair and said sandwiches, then tried to steer the conversation back to work. This was my chance to make a stand. I stopped the meeting and forced an introspective dissection of the problem. I presented the arguments above, but I was outranked and outnumbered and again, I lost.

When I got home that night I was visibly dejected. I breathed heavier than normal. I was short with my wife. Finally, she asked what was the matter and I told her about the discussion, the internet vote, the follow up discussion and how unjust the entire universe was that all of these successful people could be so wrong about an incredibly basic fact and use it to oppress me.

Then she said she was on team sandwich as well.

Bitch.

I love my wife. And I know my wife. She played division 1 rugby at UCLA. As a fullback, it was her job to tackle women up to twice her size (literally) running full speed through her to try and score, so backing down wasn't exactly her thing. She's also not prone to high stakes gambling so I threw down the gauntlet, for our standard $5 wager. Formal events and events already on the calendar aside, she could only eat sandwiches and I could only eat pizza until one of us quit.

The chorus of trolls bellows loudly at the stakes. The stakes are simple. I used to gamble a ton. I once lost over two hundred dollars in a dice game in a kitchen in riverside the same week I won over two thousand at poker in an Indian casino out in the desert. I've sat in one seat for twenty-six hours playing no-limit hold 'em three days after spending a week in the hospital for a non-gambling related health problem. I understand what it means to gamble. Winning five bucks from someone as cheap as my wife was such a better value than doubling down on a soft seventeen or going all in preflop with pocket kings or any other gambling trope we've all done to say we've done it.

Then we had to decide for the purposes of the bet, what constituted a pizza and a sandwich. For this to work we had to make certain ground rules and establish a sort of working definition in case something fell in between the definitely yes and definitely not lists. Unfortunately, we asked the internet again here and I had to sort through dozens of people on team sandwich offer sandwich advice through my Facebook page to my wife, each one beginning with a condemnation of team pizza.

As an example of how awful the internet is, two of my friends on team sandwich even got into an argument about whether a hamburger was a sandwich. It is a sandwich. Look at it. That was the keystone to this bet. You know in your heart of hearts what a sandwich is and what a sandwich isn't, but just to be safe we set out ground rules. A sandwich is something between two pieces of bread. You must eat it as a sandwich. Don't do anything stupid like put a crouton on each side of a giant chicken breast and call that a sandwich, but if you wanted to put a bunch of croutons inside of a baguette that would work because that is in the true spirit of the sandwich!

As far as what is pizza, it's fairly obvious. At this point I realized I should've made the sandwich vs. pie bet, as pizza is a type of pie, but it was too late. And if we're being completely honest, there are only a couple pies I really enjoy: pizza, oreo, peach, pecan and pineapple, and aside from pizza I only eat pie on two days each year: Thanksgiving and Fourth of July, so the fact that I suddenly couldn't crush a rhubarb in one sitting wasn't too devastating, but I could tell dessert would be a challenge.

Rules, stakes, duration and qualifications agreed upon, we each placed five dollars each in escrow on our bedroom tv stand and went to bed, not knowing how long the adventure we were embarking upon would last, nor how it would affect our relationship, social lives and bodies, but also not caring. For now, it was about pizza and sandwiches and honor.

2. "THE BET."

We started the bet on a Tuesday. I don't know why. I know we had a reason, but I can't remember it. We had ramen on Monday night from a cash-only spot a couple miles away from home as our last meal before the bet.

The best ramen is cash only. That's a fake hot take - a hot fake, because I've had ramen like, three times when it wasn't from a steaming-hot Styrofoam container. My ramen experience however, does include a habit I rocked freshman year of college that ran parallel to my foray into chewing tobacco. The two terribly unhealthy habits met in perfect synergy once when I repurposed an instant ramen cup full of dip-spit by heating it in the microwave and dumping it off a third-floor balcony. It was well below freezing at that particular time of winter and my scientific hypothesis was that dip-spitsicles would form before hitting the ground. When that obviously didn't work, and I found little white hairs growing under my tongue, I quit both habits. Point is, we started on a Tuesday.

Day one, I skipped breakfast. That was the plan: skip breakfast. I read an article on the internet that called it intermittent fasting, but none of the uninformed troglodytes around me would allow for that terminology so I called it skipping breakfast. Really though, it was so much more. I stopped all calorie consumption at ten pm and trained hard from one to two pm before eating the next day, and then trained again from eight to nine pm before eating again before ten. If that's not fasting, fine. Enjoy your sandwiches you semantic monsters.

17

I skipped breakfast and trained from one to two pm. I went for a run around the park across from work. At the time, my salary was not enough for a luxurious gym membership. This meant I had to change in the bathroom at work. I put my work clothes over my running clothes, chug a bunch of branch chain amino acids, drive across the street to the park, strip down to the running gear under my work clothes, run, cool off, put my work clothes back over my sweaty running clothes, go back to the bathroom at work and change back into my work clothes before going back to work. I did not shower. I spent a lot of money on baby powder and eau de toilet.

I was still sweating when I walked into the cafe at work. There were three dining options plus the occasional food truck. All of them offer deli sandwiches and there's always a line, but the pizza counter is always ready to serve. That shows you what kind of dumb jerks I work with; they'd rather wait in line for sandwiches than have better food right away. That doesn't make any sense to me. In retrospect though, once these idiots realize how much of their lives they've wasted in line for sandwiches when they could've been eating pizza instead, they'll probably fuck up the pizza market and I'll have to spend more money to get my fix.

Pre-pizza bet I was good for the pizza combo two to three times a week. It's a good deal if you break it down: two slices, a side and a drink you could swap for another side. You can have a half pound side salad and a banana along with your two slices and be very full for like six bucks. That was the only thing I've ever purchased at that pizza counter, so when I walked in still sweating, went about my normal routine, and sat down on the patio with food in hand, I quickly realized the banana and the chicken salad were both useless to me.

It was the first official meal of the bet. I had to nail it. Wasting food is personally disgusting to me on many levels, so I go out of my way to avoid it. I go a long way out of my way to avoid it. How far out of my way do I go to avoid wasting food? Pepperoni pizza with boiled chicken, spinach, onions, oil, vinegar, and banana. That's right. Rather than disregard the non-pizza items, I dumped it on my pizza. And I'm glad I did it. It was the worst pizza I've ever had (though for the record: even bad pizza is better than great

18

sandwiches), so I had to force it down, but I knew I was doing the right thing. As I was chuffing it, my boss walked by and stopped.

"Are you eating a pizza with banana and a salad on it?" he asked, grinning.

"I am."

"Is this part of the bet?"

"Yeah. this is the first meal, actually."

"It looks gross."

"It's not optimal."

"Good luck," and he walked off; probably to get a sandwich. It was exactly then - meal one day one of the bet, that I knew I was going to win. Not because of the obvious superiority of pizza over sandwiches, but because even though I was eating this pizza abomination, it still relatively palatable. If I could eat this pizza and be happy enough with it to not be put off from the whole bet, then just a small amount of planning would make things easy. It was about to be the best few weeks of my gastronomic life.

I muscled the rest of it down and a peace came over me. My entire life leading up until that day, eating pizza was going to be my best meal of the day, because it was pizza and you're not allowed to have pizza again right after it. But this day, the first day of the pizza bet, the bad pizza I had was still pizza, and I knew two things: I would have pizza again for dinner, which was an awesome thought, and it would be so much better than the pizza I had for lunch.

All the times I'd had pizza twice in a day in my pre-pizza-bet life were often a case of finishing the lunch pie for dinner, also known as leftovers. It was better the first time because of freshness, but also because the second pizza meal on those days was tinged with a hint of sadness and failure. With each bite I could hear society asking aloud, "Pizza again, Greg? That's fucking pathetic." Society would sneer no more. Now that it was part of a good ole fashioned American prop bet, society would just stand and applaud and shed a single tear for the bravery and courage I was displaying. I was taking it to the sandwich crowd one slice at a time!

The second meal of the day went over well. I've got pizza spots all over town from the time I tried to find the best slice in Los Angeles and one of them is mulberry street pizza, which is directly on my way home from work. Since there's two locations in the San Fernando valley where I live, it doesn't matter which way I take home, one will be on the way. Location, location, location. I didn't need to, but I grabbed a whole pie at Mulberry Street. Three reasons: it's cheaper than slices, I'd need more pizza no matter what, and this was not a calorie counting diet, so I could technically have however much I wanted. Everyone thinks pizza is bad for you, but the secret is: pizza is good for you. Too much pizza is bad for you, there's a difference.

The real reason we eat too much pizza is because we know that society won't abide us having it as often we'd like. We load up whenever the pizza comes around, devouring as much as we can to keep our soul happy until the next time. But if you're smack-dab in the middle of a pizza bet and the next time you get pizza is at the next meal, you can really pace yourself. Your life is only pizza and you're finally living the way you should -- the way you've always wanted. It's as if you died and went to pizza heaven and a light shone on every meal you had ever wanted, and it was all pizza, and it was glorious.

The next day at work, I knew I needed a better plan. On the upside, I knew of pizza places all over town. Unfortunately, there weren't enough near the office that could lure me away from the convenience of a decent spot just downstairs. Which is to say the marginal benefit of traveling to the slice was not equal to the marginal cost of getting that slice. Additionally, the pizza at the office was not worth the ala carte price and one chicken, onion, spinach, oil, vinegar, banana, pepperoni pizza was enough, and I was not about to waste food. So, I had to find something decent enough in close enough proximity and cheap enough to make it worth my while.

"There should be an app!" I said. "Like Weedmaps, but for pizza!" I googled my brilliant idea, "Weedmaps but pizza", and found the pizza map app. I should've been heartbroken that my amazing billion-dollar idea was already a thing, but instead I was just stoked to have an app to help me find pizza wherever I was whenever I was there!

The app sucked, and I ended up using yelp instead.

From there, I stuck to a couple consistent spots unless I could recruit friends or coworkers to tag along. I only did that with the best of places. That way, it became a very social experience. Plus, I could tell the story of the bet and the diet, which also raised the stakes. The more people knew about the bet, the less likely I was to bail. And if they were a part of it, up close and in person, it felt like I had a team of support.

It was the only time in my life where people would invite me to lunch consistently. The Hollywood stereotype is that everyone just bumps into each other and says "lunch?" and then they do it. My experience is that everyone will agree to lunch, but I'm always the one to suggest it. I guess I should take the hint. Nobody ever says no, though, so I can't be too repulsive.

My favorite quick hitter was Little Caesar's, home of the five-dollar hot and ready pizza. You just can't beat five dollars and no waiting for a whole pizza! I've been eating Little Caesar's since I can remember. I eat it so much I gave it a nickname: Lil C's. Lil C's has fun with pizza. The week the pizza bet started I was delighted for their latest experiment, the pretzel pizza. The crust was pretzeled, brushed with a baking soda mixture I bet, and then salted out of the oven. The sauce wasn't sauce, it was liquid cheese like the kind you'd dip a pretzel in, and the cheese and pepperoni were just as tasty and salty as the crust. something that the other big pizza chains wouldn't try because they think they're real pizza and pretend to have standards, but they don't, and they over-charge. Lil C's on the other hand understands their place in the world and fills it completely with charm and grace. The pretzel pizza exemplifies the true glory of pizza, in a way that other experimental pizzas don't because they're too busy hiring fancy chefs and charging hella money for what is essentially peasant food. No, I don't want your large, melted blocks of mozzarella for twelve additional dollars. Shred it like you said you could on your resume when you got hired here, fancy pizza man.

Four days in, I started to feel strange. Like a body-wide tingling that wouldn't fade until lunchtime. I swatted a fly out of midair like it was flying in slow motion. I called a friend to tell him about it. He mocked me outright, asked why I didn't use chopsticks. My brain was full of pizza. The way a man with a hammer sees everything as a nail, my brain only thought of pizza. My new-found special power was seeing the world in slow motion. My conversational skills however, couldn't keep up, and I began to uncontrollably think out loud.

"Would chopsticks be an effective or even a reasonable pizza delivery device?" The thinking was quick, and decisive, despite the cheese and sauce powered synapses. "No. Under no circumstances should pizza be consumed with chopsticks. Not even if they're cute little baby pizzas or little pizza rolls. Even if you studied abroad in japan for a summer and acquired transitions lenses along with a ponytail and keep manga on their coffee tables like, 'what these old things?' It's just not practical."

"What?" he said.

"What?" I said back. I think I blacked out.

"I meant to kill the fly. Like karate kid. Daniel Russo."

"Oh. nah." And we waited a couple seconds before hanging up. Guys are weird.

Saturday of week one, less than 24-hours after my chopstick-verdict, was our first asterisk day. A wedding. When we came to terms of the bet we agreed that it could not interfere with actual real life. Therefore, events that were worthy of being put on a calendar: weddings, funerals, baptisms, bar mitzvahs, were asterisks. If some jerk came up to us at our event for which we went through the trouble of making and sending invitations and planning and all that, and they asked us for two special considerations in order to stay on board with a five-dollar bet, we'd probably just ask them to leave, making sure to pick up a gift registry on the way out. Asking that could and should jeopardize friendships and careers. It would be completely unacceptable and though we are quite selfish, we knew better.

The rules for these events were simple. For the duration of the event, the bet was off. The wedding was a fantastic affair at a big hotel in downtown. It was a bit later than what most people would consider a late lunch time, but since my wife and I are habitual late eaters, it was just lunch time. Rather than doubling up, having lunch at two and then again at three-thirty, we skipped lunch. That doesn't mean we weren't late, because we were incredibly late. We are always late to everything. It has nothing to do with pizza or sandwiches, it's just who we are. We were so late, we arrived during the cocktail hour after the ceremony. We spent the first ten minutes hovering over the appetizers stuffing our faces, concocting a lie about how gorgeous the ceremony was.

Luckily thanks to a lack of mutual friends with the bride and groom and our general unapproachableness, we didn't have to lie to anyone. This meant we weren't embarrassed when the whole room was invited in to start the ceremony.

It turns out that even though this was a very fancy and immaculately planned and executed wedding, it fell into the same trap as every other wedding in the history of weddings: it was late. The major difference between this one and less fancy weddings was that this wedding's tardiness was planned for and catered. Naturally, we believed this was a post-ceremony cocktail hour, but it was simply pre-ceremony hors d'oeuvres.

No pizzas were mentioned until dinner when the bride and groom swung by to say hello and teed us up to the rest of the table. Everyone who heard about the bet instantly chose a side and unless it was pizza they were wrong.

We don't dance at weddings so unless I'm getting wrecked, we leave at a reasonable hour. Also, my wife had a work soccer tournament early the next morning. With the early morning promised and the probable lack of shade common at soccer fields, I felt like it would be an awful place to bring a hangover no matter what food I brought along to ease the pain. Now that I think about it, even when I do get wrecked, we leave at a reasonable hour. I've still yet to find that sweet spot between teetotalism and slurring my favorite shoe brands for different running surfaces to the busboy when he asks if he can fill my water glass again.

The soccer tournament was everything I thought it would be: early, hot and entirely devoid of pizza. It was at the StubHub center and guests could purchase a box lunch in the luxury suite, but it was a sandwich and a bag of chips, so I opted to stick to beer which was conveniently for sale. Being drunk in the sun all day is fine, and in fact quite pleasant; the absolute opposite side of the misery spectrum from being hungover in the sun which ranks just above having to eat nothing but sandwiches for any longer than three meals. The memory from the rest of that day is mostly just beer and black but not because I blacked out, which I definitely did not, but because it was quite unremarkable. I had a milkshake on the way home though, which was delicious and since it was a drink, it was totally legit.

That night I slept harder than I had in years. Normally I go to bed around eleven and lie there for a while before finally finding sleep around midnight. I wake up at four for a quick bathroom break, toss and turn for twenty minutes, then wake up again at seven for another pee, then toss and turn for forty minutes before resetting my alarm from eight to eight thirty and then stew and half-sleep until then, snooze twice and then hurry in to work. But after a week on an exclusive pizza diet, I would drop off to sleep almost immediately. I'd blink and wake up at five to pee and then drop right back to sleep until my alarm went off at eight. No snooze needed. Just pop right up and get going feeling rested and excited for a day of pizza. There was no reason to go back to sleep and dream of pizza when I could be awake and live that dream.

At this point, early in the bet, I had lost two pounds and could see glimpses of the future. I didn't see lottery tickets or anything, but I could predict where things would be in space and when. It was just an overwhelming feeling of clarity. Looking back, that was probably just a pizza fueled manic fugue state.

3. "THE MAGIC BULLET."

I read a fair number of books that could be considered the self-help or self-improvement kind. I also read a lot of non-fiction and history books. If you look at my amazon orders, my favorites are narrative memoirs covering hidden diet secrets and fountains of youth and magic cure all's are. It's simple: everyone wants the easy path to be great. "Maybe it's in this book. Though it was definitely not in the last one, or the one before that, or everyone before that. This is the one!"

That rationale is a cycle I've seen so many times in poker rooms and around craps tables in Indian casinos. Folks who had no business gambling, who should be at work, but instead they're sixteen hours deep with their fixed incomes on the table. Repeatedly they would lose because that's the business of casinos. That should not be the business of self-help.

It is, unfortunately the business of self-help. If any of these fucking books worked, it'd be the last book you bought. There is no secret to success. We all know how to lose weight. We all know how to be a lawyer or a doctor too. The secret to losing weight or your medical or juris doctorate degree is a specific regimen of focused work. The hard part isn't knowing what to do, it's doing it.

This is why eight weeks into every program I pick out of a self-help book, I give up. "I've been eating only green things for two months and I haven't been to the Olympics once, I must be doing something wrong, I'm the worst!" Or something like that. I've tried a hundred diets and I've never once been an elite athlete, why are all these elite athletes hocking diets? Because dumb fucks like me buy them.

The fact remains. If you're an elite athlete, it doesn't matter what you do, what you eat, what you wear, you'll be an elite athlete. I've spent a year swimming four days a week and jumped in the pool with my best friend who swam and played water polo in high school and plays inner tube water polo between business trips and sales calls and was absolutely trounced by him in what he thought were warmups.

There might be some science behind lifetime total training volume or something, or there might not be. It could just be psychological. I am not a scientist, so I couldn't tell you. I lifted weights three times a week for six months and still get out lifted by women half my bodyweight regularly. Should I wear women's clothing and grow my hair out? No. that's a silly thing to try. They have more experience, their bodies have different levers, and I'm just a dork with a gym membership. It's not the clothing or the hair style, it's the athlete or the author.

So why would we think that reading a book about a different person's diet would work any differently than the clothing they choose or the hair style they prefer? You can put the same gas in a car and a lawnmower and I'll tell you from my sofa, with a beer in my hand, which one can cut grass better and which one will run a faster quarter mile. My point is, we are all machines who do what we have been designed to do, and if you're not an elite athlete, changing something as superficial as fuel isn't going to make you one. What makes you one is how much work you've put in, how much time you've consistently put that work in and how much success you have had because of that work over that time.

That said, eat pizza and you will lose weight and be a better person. If you don't, then you've obviously done something terribly wrong and should buy another couple copies of this book. And also send me some dr. pepper. Can't say it will help me lose weight but it's tasty.

4. "SKYDIVE."

Collere is expensive, so I knew my freshman year that I wanted to be an RA (resident advisor: a person who's a year older but is somehow in control of your bedtime). One, it was a pretty sweet job, and two, they paid for your room and board. In addition to that, living on campus as you're forced to do for your job makes your estimated cost of attendance extremely high which will bump up your partial need-based scholarship. In my case, being an RA for two years and making a hundred to a hundred and fifty dollars per month, the very little extra money left over after tuition and parking and health insurance and all the other nonsense was extremely helpful.

The downside to being an RA was not being able to have alcohol in my room or throw a party or even be drunk at home lest there was an emergency and I had to go to work. I say downside, but it was just a tradeoff, because there were incredible perks to being an RA. The work was incredibly fulfilling. I was basically just mentoring a group of people in my peer group while living with them and giving them the extra knowledge they would need to protect themselves from life and if life got out of control, provide the tools and support they might need to prevail, which I would do anyway. My free room and board also included fourteen meals per week in the residential restaurants (fancy name for cafeteria). That boiled down to two all you can eat buffets per day. Another downside was sometimes shit went down and you'd have to work insane hours on short or no notice, like the time the cafeteria burnt down after dinner one night and we worked from ten pm to ten am with no breaks. They made up for it when they rebuilt the cafeteria, though, and added a pizza station which was as awesome as it sounds.

Having been out from under my parents' roof for four years and never having had a beer at my desk or in my shower or on my toilet like all of my friends had in their own apartments was kind of a letdown I had never even slept in my own bed drunk (this is mostly a lie, but in case my old bosses read this, it's absolutely true.). I wanted those experiences because they were experiences my peer group would have and I did not want them with a dumb office job harshing my mell. Which is a long way of saying I took a fifth year in college to complete my college experience in an off-campus apartment.

At first, I had a job lined up at a local building supplies warehouse store. A retail associate job at the place where one would have stopped if one were working on their home. A retail associate job that would have involved wearing an orange apron. This place shall remain nameless to protect the innocent. I didn't want that job, but I knew I would need to work twenty to thirty hours a week in order to make rent and eat and have gas in my car in addition to the loan I would have to take to pay for my tuition and books.

I also was a blossoming poet and screenwriter at the time. I scored a gig at a local video rental place. A video rental place that would potentially bust a block. A video rental place that would make me wear a blue and yellow shirt, but since they didn't have long sleeve versions in stock in southern California, and since I had tattoos, I had to buy my own long sleeve shirts to wear under to cover my tattoos. That's a dumb rule, but I put up with it to stand around and talk movies with customers all day and get free rentals.

Unfortunately, the hours conflicted with each other, so I chose the video rental place, but they didn't give enough hours, so I needed another job. I complained out loud to two of my closest friends one night and they said the place where they and their third roommate worked was hiring. A pizza place. Firehouse Pizza. I was told to bring in my license and proof of auto insurance and the interview was just "hey, when can you start?" I suited up the next day. The week before I was technically between jobs, but this week I had three offers and one of them was at a pizza shop.

I had been to that pizza shop once before, after a softball game my freshman year. One of our guys, Gus, worked there and it was two blocks from the field. I was somewhat of a ringer on the team and wouldn't dare miss an opportunity to hang with a bunch of fourth and fifth years. Another ringer was my RA's boss. Neither of us thought much of it until the pitcher of beer landed right in between us and our hands touched on the handle. He was mid-twenties and in charge of my RA whose job was pretty much to make sure I didn't make poor or illegal choices, so he was doubly in charge of that. In any case, our hands touched on the handle and recoiled instantly. "I'm just a guy," he said, which meant that outside of the residence halls (fancy name for dorms) he was just a person and that stayed out there. It was my first lesson in work life balance. You're not your job, ever. Then we both got half drunk and were late to a meeting and the pizza was fantastic. And free.

I had been to Firehouse Pizza and had good memories there, which made it easier to work there. There were three shops in three different neighborhoods. Two of them were co-run by a pair of sisters and the third was their brother's. The sisters, as best I could tell got along fine, but their brother never came up. I would switch between the two shops that the sisters co-ran but never the third which was another clue that their brother was probably on the outs. I mainly worked at the one at which I wasn't hired, which meant an extra twenty bucks cash for the trouble of driving all the way across town and it wasn't taxed. That added up to an extra hundred bucks a week from five shifts at the pizza gig. This was about equal to the take home pay from fifteen hours a week at the other job, which I hated almost instantly.

It didn't take long to realize how soul-sucking it was to work at a video shop for the people who manage video shops. The gig sucked. It dragged. I was just alone for five hours a day four days a week up front while the manager schworffed taco bell in the back room watching the

THE GREAT PIZZA EXPERIMENT

security monitors and only would come out to tell me not to talk to customers too long, not to look at my phone even when the store was empty, not to watch the movie that was playing on all the screens, and even not to keep my sodas on the back shelf behind the register. I hated it and what made it worse is that we had to upsell their online thing which was trying to compete with Netflix. It was from a group of corporate minds who didn't think of it and were ill-equipped to innovate against a startup type company like Netflix. I put in my two weeks and got my next eight shifts covered and walked out. I still have the shirts though, at twenty bucks each and having never been washed, I would never throw those things away. At the very least, in twenty years I can wear one and explain to all the kids who will listen what DVDs were and the fact that we had to drive to a store to borrow them.

Aside from the tips at the pizza shop, the work was light and the company was dope. The sisters ran the place, but their dad owned it. For the first four months, I never saw him, but he was there every day. You knew he was there because when you opened the store, the oven would be hot and there would be dough mixing in the bowl and two freshly-smoked Salem Menthol cigarette butts in the ashtray. Every day, the old dude would wake up early, come to his shop, have a smoke, turn on the oven and mix up some dough, have another smoke and then bounce before we all got in to work. He was a pizza spook. Invisible but with a signature that almost made him into a miniature myth.

The first time I saw him was when I delivered him a pizza. It was a total boss move. There was name on the ticket, but no total. I went to the manager, surely it was a mistake. She laughed, told me who he was and told me to hurry. I was excited to see how the owner of a small pizza empire lived but the address on the ticket led me to a bar: The Skydive. It was right by the airport and was parachute themed, but it was also the diviest dive under the sky. Eleven in the morning on a Thursday I walked into an unairconditioned, muggy, dank, pitch black bar with a free pizza with my boss' dad's name on it. I called his name and he raised his hand. One of three people in the place aside from me, and that's when I saw him. He was unremarkable except for his Ugg boots. Dude crushed those Ugg boots. Every time I saw him from then on, he was wearing those Ugg boots.

He tipped, which was unexpected in context, but appreciated. After that day, I would try and show up early to my opening shift to hang out and smoke a cigarette with him, but even when I was there at the same time he never wanted to talk. Which is why the time I saw him stumbling home from the skydive I didn't pull over to give him a lift, but instead went back to the shop. I snitched on him to one of the troop of his grandchildren who worked in the shop with me. She rolled her eyes and left immediately to go swoop him up and take him home.

5. "THE WALL."

My family moved from New Jersey to California when I was three years old. We moved because my parents always wanted to live in California - at the beach, and my mom's sister and mother had already moved there. My mom's mom needed some assistance because she was an old widow with some health problems. My mom's sister couldn't do it all by herself, and family comes first. But to hear them tell it, they always dreamt of living at the beach, so they moved out to California which is probably true, but the timing was definitely accelerated to fit the situation. We moved to the inland empire which is as far from the beach as it sounds. To be fair, they looked in some beach towns, but the schools were terrible, so we moved to the city of trees and PHDs, Claremont. It was rad, but I still can't surf.

My mom's sister was a "TV lady." That's all we knew and looking back that's all we needed to know. Why should kids understand the subtleties of a career as an "executive producer of first run syndication and non-fiction television programs"? All we knew was she was the lady who would tickle us until we said she was our favorite aunt and take us to visit her at work on sets or control rooms. She would take us to watch movies which were always free because she had some magical card that got us all in. It was so cool. It was our favorite thing to do because it made us feel famous or whatever. Back in the day you had to look in the newspaper to see what movies were playing where and at what time. We didn't ever get the newspaper, so we would just drive to the movie theatre and chose a movie off the marquis.

There's something to be said for the concept of fifteen minutes of fame. Maybe not that everybody gets one, but everybody wants just one small instance where they feel special, like the center of attention. For some it's their wedding. For nerds it's the valedictorian speech, or for running nerds it's the packet pickup before the race, or for obstacle course racing nerds it's the post-race expo. I have lower standards, of course.

One of these trips to the movies was literally life changing. It was in the middle of the week during the summer. She came and picked me and my brother and my sister for another one of our movie runs. We probably decided on naked gun. I don't know why I think that, I just remember watching that movie with her and you'll never know the difference, anyway. The only problem was: it was around lunch time and the movie didn't start for an hour. We asked the ticket taker what was nearby to eat. She said there was a fancy sit-down Chinese place, an El Pollo Loco and a pizza place. We chose the pizza place because at the time my diet included pb&j, plain pasta, chicken nuggets, and cheese pizza.

It was called San Biagio's. The entryway was crowded with video games, the scent of smoldering tomatoes and garlic hung thick in the air. The menu board had been there for years as you could see by the lower part's gentle fade from white to yellow as you got closer to the pizza oven over which it hung. The prices of the pizzas had changed over time, the layers of tape with the prices written on them peeled at the corners betraying their impermanence. New menu items were written in sharpie on paper plates and taped to any surface - zeppole on the register, stromboli hung off the bottom of the menu board, calzones taped to the glass that guarded the slices under heat lamps.

Polaroids of the oldish man who welcomed us when we walked in hung on the wall. Each one featured a very happy family - a different one every time, sitting in the restaurant at tables full of pizza, salad bowls, and soda pitchers. The happiest person in every photo was him: the eponymous Biagio proprietor who spoke little English through a thick Sicilian accent. He took the order from behind a stained white shirt under a silly cap the color of the Italian flag, his uniform from all the photos.

Then he turned around and went about making our food while we found a table. His energy was incredible. Despite the language barrier, and the fact that he was working, he found time to leave the kitchen and goof around with us. His specialty was tapping you on the opposite shoulder from where he stood getting you to look the other direction. When he would get you, his laugh was enough to melt your embarrassment and recruit you to laugh with him, at you. I've been in comedy for almost ten years professionally, and still have not met anyone with that charisma. He could've been a cult leader but instead he made pizza.

The pizza was out of this world. It was good enough to make you shave your head, wear a robe and move into a compound. It was like none of us had ever had pizza before. The four of us - my brother, my sister and my aunt, ate a pizza that was meant to serve five. Then we ordered another and ate that. We're Italians from New Jersey. We eat pizza, and this blew us away. It was so good we joked about going back after the movie but didn't because we had to be home. Even though she was a grown up and fully in charge, our favorite aunt the babysitter still had a curfew.

We got home and did not shut up about the pizza. It was the first good pizza we'd had since we left new jersey and pizza is so fucking good that when you find good pizza you talk about it until you fall asleep. We hyped it so hard that our parents took us back the next day. They loved it too. My mom especially liked his English speckled with Italian and long pauses while he thought of the right word; just like her grandparents from the old country.

We went about once a month and there would never be leftovers. If there was pizza we were eating it, even if we were full. As a family of five we'd crush two twenty-inch pies and I have little doubt that we could have completely destrominated a fifth if we could have afforded it. It was amazing pizza and you get what you pay for. The premium pie comes at a premium price and while it was worth it, cash wasn't always our strong suit, so we made due. I say made due like we weren't driving two towns over for expensive pizza like a bourgeois family of east coast transplants in the suburbs of Los Angeles, maybe I'm just bitter we didn't have five pizzas.

My Dad's sister came to visit from new jersey. We were so stoked to show her we had good pizza that we convinced her to take us. Except we were all kids. We didn't know where it was. She was from New Jersey, so she didn't know where it was, either and this was very much pre-internet. We knew it was on mountain avenue, but we lived at the foot of the San Gabriel Mountains. There are four mountain avenues in a twenty-minute radius, so after driving the length of the first two we gave up and got Round Table, a premium regional pizza chain that was our usual first choice when guests came to town or other fancy pizza occasions. She told our parents about our mishap and they took us all the next night. Best week ever and my dad's sister liked it so much that she told the rest of their jersey family about it so every time they visited they requested it. Years between visits and my cousin's first words after landing every time would be 'San Biagi's."

As with all regulars we learned the rhythm of the place. We learned the employees' names - they were all his kids, so we were essentially just hanging out with his family. We learned that sometimes he'd leave them in charge and on those days the pizza would be different. We learned he was a Yankees fan and those games would always be on. We learned that the non-pizza foods were comparably amazing and should not be skipped in favor of pizza. Most importantly, we learned that if you're going to show up after two hours before closing on a Sunday night you should take it to go. We learned that the hard way after a couple consecutive grumpy hurried experiences and then we finally pieced it together. We were officially regulars.

Then on my fourteenth birthday, it happened. It was just an ordinary night - family dining at the long table near the jukebox. We sat while my parents ordered and after the pitchers of soda and salads came out, the pizzas followed. Everything we ordered was on the table but when Biagio left the table after his customary comedy bits, went behind the counter and came back with a polaroid camera. This was it. We were getting made.

I see it in slow motion in my memory, his jowly laugh, his free hand instructing us to scroonch in closer, the flash, more laughing as the picture printed, the polaroid shake, and then more laughter as we passed the picture around the table. He took it and put it on the wall behind the sticker machine.

The last time I remember seeing it was three years after it was taken, on my seventeenth birthday when I was really stoned and pretended to be very interested in the stickers, so nobody would know I was high, not really considering that a seventeen-year-old enthralled by shiny stickers in a shit vending machine was obviously on drugs. I've never been a regular anywhere else in my entire life until the pizza bet gave me that gift at my local Neapolitan express joint. But even then, all that Neapolitan place did was recognize me, they didn't make me and my entire family polaroid famous immortals like San Biagio.

6. "EXPERIMENTS."

Week two of the pizza bet started off great. Lighter weight and better rest made me very happy to be alive. One thing pizza couldn't do though, was cure my road rage. I have a horrendous commute. I have the worst commute on earth. I have a commute so bad it wins awards for badness. I have a commute so bad that rich people have started chartering helicopters to get around it. I drive on the 405 freeway in Los Angeles, California.

The freeway is fine. It's wide, it's fast, it only has one curve that generates actual traffic. There's a groaner joke that goes "don't get on the four oh five between four oh five and four oh five," which sounds hilarious but the times aren't accurate if they're am and pm, even worse if it's pm and am, and worse still if it's am and am or pm and pm because that's just "don't get on the four oh five," which is dumb advice because all the side streets are jam packed. Los Angeles is full, stay where you are.

I try and cope with the stress by doing things for myself that will release the tension. I will put hexes on drivers doing things that upset me - which is just saying the word "hex!" and shooting my eyes wide at their car. I'll flip people off below the window, so they can't see, or just say "flipping you off!" as they drive past me, or I drive past them. Mostly though, I just get angry and yell things that don't help at all like "move the fuck up dumbshit!" The rage is so powerful it's pizza proof. It's the only thing in my life that did not improve one bit for the entirety of The Great Pizza Experiment, but with everything else being perfect, I had time to work on this.

I was still pretty wound up from the stress of my former pizza-rationed life. I needed to relax. I needed to find something that would slow me down. I considered smoking pot before work, but I liked my job and if there was one thing that could get you fired easily and ruin your career, it was drugs. I wondered if there was a way to slow myself down to the new speed of mi pizza vida by using pizza. Cooking the pizza was the obvious solution. My family and I made pizza growing up and I spent a year in the kitchen of a busy pizza restaurant, so it wouldn't be that difficult, but it would slow me down and connect me with the food more. I had some classic recipes, some avant-garde and some short cut recipes.

The first one I tried was just an ordinary dough with marinara and cheese. It was great but filling, and I made a couple, so I could survive on leftovers. The best part about leftover pizza is that it's pizza. The worst part is storing it. Pizzas normally come in boxes and if your refrigerator can fit it, the pizzas will stay in the box until you run out of pizza. In college, I had a job where I was on call for one weekend a month, and on those weekends, I would order two extra-large pizzas, hope the phone wouldn't ring and play online poker in my bedroom only leaving for soda or softball. Those pizzas would stay in their boxes until piece by piece, they were gone.

When I was at the pizza shop I spent a lot of time making the boxes that serve as adequate and preferred storage pieces for food items. They come in big flat bundles wrapped in plastic and live on the kitchen floor until the plastic comes off, then they live on shelves and on top of refrigerators until they're folded into boxes and filled with pizza and sent to the customer. They're origami. They absorb fluids and odors. They're full of holes. If you were to store pizza ingredients in pizza boxes in a pizza restaurant, that restaurant would be closed by the health department. Pizza boxes are a terrible place for food. You'd be better off storing pizza on a plate than in a pizza box.

When I had an entire leftover pizza on that night I decided to start cooking, I was incredibly stoked to pick up a box that I hadn't taken out to the dumpster yet and upcycle it. If a pizza box is a poor place to store food, a used pizza box that has been empty leaning against a garbage can for a day or two could be the worst place to food. I thought I was MacGyver for wrapping my pizza in trash and putting it into the fridge. Most of the pizzas I made that survived the first night went into old pizza boxes I picked up off the floor and I was super proud of myself until writing these last two paragraphs. I survived though so it's clearly not the worst idea.

The next pizza I made was a keto-pizza. I wasn't doing the keto diet, but the keto-pizza had the benefit of a different crust than normal bread. The crust was made of cheese, cream cheese, and maybe an egg. It was baked, sauced, topped and baked again. It was super crispy but also the most filling pizza slice for slice that I have ever had. It was more filling even than Chicago style pizza, which is a feat because that stuff is basically a salty molten brick. With all that cheese in the everything, the keto pizza needed some help.

Toppings are a controversial subject for some. I use them sparingly and conventionally, with the exception of pineapple which I love. That is somehow a hot take, but I feel comfortable discussing it because you already bought the book. I feel the same way about ranch that some people feel about pineapple. Ranch doesn't belong on pizza. I don't even know what ranch is, but it is some white people shit. And I say that in a way that in no uncertain terms accuses a wide swath of mashed-potato-loving, plain-hot-dog-eating, steak-sauce needing people of having a daft palate. Yes, the group of people who made IPAs the only beer style you can find at too many bars and stores, are probably the same group who invented ranch on pizza and I am personally offended by their existence.

I had some tomato plants, but a lot of the buds didn't make fruit and most of the ones that did ended up either getting wrecked by squirrels sampling the unripe tomatoes, get grossed out and leave it, or split open due to overwatering and over-fertilizing. I had two bushes and watered them every day before work for months and all I got were three golf-ball sized tomatoes. I got tomatoes, but not enough for the time spent. With a hose and a proper yard, I could keep ten plants with the same effort and fully plan on doing so if I ever get a proper yard. In any case, the keto pizza needed some help being less brickish and pizzas can only hold so much sauce, and the tiny tomatoes - Roma tomatoes should be the size of baseballs at least - were begging for a purpose. So, I sliced them up and tossed them onto my next keto pizza.

Holy shit. These things tasted like a completely different thing I had never had ever before in my entire life. I don't know how else to describe it but the flavor in those home-grown tomatoes was so different from anything I had ever eaten before including tomatoes. I felt cheated out of an entire life of flavor. I was inspired. I was mystified. If this was what tomatoes taste like, what other things had been hidden from me? Every time I said, "this tastes like tomatoes," my entire life I was lying. Incredible. I vowed to go to farmers market every week, to keep that flavor in my life, to move out of the city and grow tomatoes professionally, to reveal the true nature of taste to my fellow man. In that moment, my life was changed. I mean, it changed back to normal the next moment, but at least I knew what tomatoes really taste like. I did go to one farmers market a few months later, but I ended up forgetting tomatoes and buying honey for a home brew I was making. Oh well.

In addition to the tomato plants, I was growing basil. Basil's yield was a lot more in line with the effort it took to grow. I had so much fresh basil at all times that I started making pesto like it was going out of style. Pesto on a pizza is a special thing. I make pesto with walnuts instead of pine nuts because pine nuts are expensive as hell. I also use way too much garlic because garlic is delicious. And apparently, I make pesto without cheese, as many of the recipes I've come across add grated cheese to the oil, nut, herb mix. In any case, it was more popular than marinara as a sauce during The Great Pizza Experiment because it scaled better to individual pizzas than my tomato sauce recipe did, and it was less common at stores. If I absolutely needed the red sauce, I could easily obtain it in local stores.

The last experiment I performed was the cauliflower crust pizza. This one uses riced cauliflower, cheese and eggs as its crust that you bake, sauce, top and re-bake. It's a little tougher to nail than the ordinary dough and even the keto-pizza crust. It's got a lot of water in it and it tastes decidedly vegetably, so it wasn't my favorite until I burnt one, or so I thought. What I did was basically fry the cauliflower and make it delicious. It was such a pain to make, though, that I rarely put out the effort.

The alt crusts and sauces and toppings really helped shake things up which is extremely important, as too much of the same for too long is boring, even if that thing is amazing. This is why you see ultra-rich dudes wrap their Lamborghinis in chrome vinyl. This fact started to become apparent around day ten of the pizza bet.

Despite the absolute unending pleasure of eating so much pizza and not wasting time with any garbage, consuming the bulk of your calories from cheese has some repercussions. It goes in liquid, but it solidifies back up once it is in. ten days of gut bricks were floating down my river and I wouldn't call it a log jam, but it certainly was not comfortable in the slightest.

After ten days of eating no breakfast, pizza for lunch, pizza for dinner and pizza for snacks, the uncomfortableness in my gut was starting to stack up. Sometimes at lunch I'd get full after a comically small amount of pizza. It was a bummer, a devil's bargain. I could eat as much pizza as my heart desired, but my stomach was always full. It was torture. Worse than the internal limits on pizza consumption were the general effects of having cement for guts. It was truly uncomfortable. It was sometimes dangerous.

I am very physically active. I grew up normal enough, but in high school I started to get very fat, eventually exceeding our family scale's three-hundred-pound limit well before I turned it around by moving to college and being forced to walk everywhere. I bet I was in the three ten to three twenty-five range. In any case. A little activity got me a little result. Then I started playing intramural softball and saw more results. I plateaued at an above average weight until I was hospitalized and diagnosed with ulcerative colitis. When I was released from the hospital, I was underweight for the first time since junior high school and I definitely enjoyed the benefits that being not fat afforded me.

Once I got healthy again, some of the weight came back. I was not obese, but I was back to being just overweight enough to make me self-conscious. Then I was out of college and working full time and my friend asked me to be a groomsman at his wedding. The thought of being forever captured in their wedding photos that they'd show their grandkids as a fat guy was horrifying. I started running that day. A mile every other day at first. Then two. Then three and four and then running to the pool and swimming and lifting weights and hiking and anything I could do to work up a sweat. I was so addicted physical exertion that I would volunteer myself for yard work at my friends' houses in the suburbs. They all paid in my two favorite things: beer and pizza.

By the time The Great Pizza Experiment started I had logged multiple 5k and 10k races, Tough Mudders, Spartan races, multiple ten-thousand-foot mountain peaks (the tallest within a four-hour drive) Multiple day backpacking trips deep into the backcountry, too many half marathons to count, a couple marathons and even a 50k ultramarathon were in there too. To have this many and this variety of distances under your belt you needed to have a passion for exercise. This all pizza diet wasn't making it impossible for me to exercise but it was stealing the joy of it. There's two parts to exercise, the work and the endorphins. The work is hard, the endorphins balance that out. You know what kills endorphins? Fear of shitting your pants. Runner's trots are a risk when you go out for any run, but when you have packed your gut with cheese and are one to two days behind your normal schedule, you're literally carrying a bomb around in your shorts and it could go off at any time, and don't get me started on back squats!

The pizza bet was meant to be fun and firing a high velocity doodie brick into your boxer briefs on your lunch break at the office gym is probably the farthest thing from fun you could get. That's if it stayed in your boxer briefs; those things are pretty flimsy and if it's getting past your panic racked butthole, then that thin bit of cotton doesn't stand a chance. Let me be clear, I didn't poop myself on this diet, but I had before. I have looked into the abyss of mass accidental discharge and did not like what I saw and did not want to risk it again. For this reason, and after careful consideration of the rules of the bet and the diet, I started replacing dinner with a protein smoothie. This is another stopping point for dickfaces who hate life, telling me that it doesn't count. It does. It simply does. The same diet I drank a ton of beer, probably five milkshakes per week, a gallon or two of water every day and none of that caused concern with the rules, why is a smoothie any different? I have an answer, it's because you are angry you haven't had pizza yet today. Go have a slice, you get really troll-y when you're hungry.

The smoothies helped a lot. I could exercise twice a day like I've always wanted to and not worry about detonating a shit nuke any more than any other day. To be very clear I'm at an elevated risk for self-shitting because of the same ulcerative colitis that I was diagnosed with, so the diet made things worse than they already were and had to be hacked. The knowledge that I could house an entire pie for lunch with no consequences was better than not spending every moment in fear of pooping myself because that's already my everyday life. This was just that normal life but with pizza. It was like being in love.

The last day of the second week there was a baby shower for a friend of ours. As the rules stated, calendar worthy events were considered days off, so my wife was very much looking forward to this break from sandwiches. I was looking forward to it as well, but for very different reasons: I just like people. We got to the shower, late, of course but reasonably late for a big town like Los Angeles. Everyone was excited to talk to us about our bet as I share heavily on social media. My girlfriend had skipped breakfast and went right for the party food: chips and crackers had no reasonable sandwich facsimile, so she was going hard as fuck on them. I caught up with folks, then cruised past the food table on my way to the beer. I had to have something as I was just coming off a fast, so unless I wanted to be luggage by lunch, I would need to eat.

I stood in front of the food table, on my day off of the dang bet, free from any limitations. I could eat anything I wanted. It was this moment that confirmed I had the right answer to the original question. I could eat anything I wanted, and I chose pizza. There were kids at the party, and their palates did not yet have a taste for the classy food my girlfriend was hammering, the sushi, the crudité, the salads, the cured meats and cheese platters and all that other party stuff, so there was pizza at the party. It was nothing special, just some frozen oven pizza. I could eat anything I wanted, and I chose pizza. It was the pizza that all the kids had to share so the adults could have their adult food. I had a choice to eat food provided for me, or to indulge, and potentially deprive a child of sustenance by eating the only thing they could eat, and I chose the latter. I had transcended the bet.

Everyone knew the rules of the bet and couldn't believe it. "It's your cheat day," they would say, "why are you eating pizza?"

"It's a free day, yes," I would answer, "all that means is I can eat whatever I want, and I want pizza."

"DAMN!" they would say and look right at my girlfriend and her bag of veggies or other non-sandwich food choice, and she would shrug like it didn't faze her, but we had been together seven years at this point and I knew it was cleaving into her soul. This is the day she began to break. The next morning was the first day of the third week on the pizza bet. I was 6.8 pounds lighter than day 1, generally cheerful, and I could hear animals' thoughts when I touched them.

7. "THE PROMOTION."

When I started The Great Pizza Experiment, I had been at my job for 2 years. The job was a junior position that I was barely qualified for when I started, but I was a quick learner and had all of the skill and abilities necessary to succeed. I had graduated in my mind to being underemployed. I was taking meetings with other companies which was actually super convenient because I was out every day at lunch getting pizza from somewhere, so nobody even missed me.

After a couple weeks of good meetings I could tell I was close to an offer from a vendor with whom our company did a ton of work and both leadership teams were very close professionally and personally as is often the case in our wing of the entertainment industry. I was feeling very good. Walking around weightless and full of pizza I glided everywhere I went and I glowed, plus I was close to getting the first promotion I had ever received, even if it was at a different company it still would've been a first. Mostly it was the pizza.

As I was gliding past my boss' boss' office the door opened and my boss' eyes lit up as if to say "there you are! I was just about to go get you!" he waved me in. it was crowded in there. My boss and a couple other people on his level, all of whom oversaw the creative content our group put out, and their boss behind his desk greeted me heartily as I entered. Everyone was incredibly happy to see me.

I had never been promoted before. In my head, promotions were things like this - a group of higher ups in a room call in the plebe and give him the good news. Everyone laughs and pats you on the back and then you sign some papers, there's more laughing and congratulating and then it's over. It wouldn't be unlike the ceremony to enter the Cosa Nostra. One day you aren't, then you get sent for, then you do this thing and then you are. Boom. this was it. This was the New Jersey basement in which my hand would be cut so my blood could mix with candle wax on a picture of a saint. They had heard I was out trying to join another crew and they wanted to make me an offer I couldn't refuse.

There was a buzz in the room. As we settled they motioned for me to have a seat. "So, Greg. They tell me--" oh here we go! The vendor snitched on me during some sort of executive golf outing and all it took for my bosses to see the light was someone else to notice my level of talent. I should've taken all those meetings way sooner. I left so much money on the table! I could've been promoted a year ago!

"They tell me you've eaten nothing but pizza for the past three weeks?"

Oh. fuck. Pizza. This is about pizza. I'm not being validated for years of loyalty, hard work, and creative brilliance, I'm being interrogated about my diet.

"Isn't that too much cheese? Doesn't that lock you up?"

Yeah. my bowel movements are being discussed openly in my boss' boss' office. Not mine specifically but the nondescript you, the editorial you. Which was me. The you who if they eat too much cheese and not enough fiber like for example if hypothetically you were only to consume pizza which you would do if you had eaten nothing but pizza for the past three weeks, which was me, which I had, but my boss' boss surely wouldn't want to discuss a specific employee's bowel movements with this many witnesses, would he?

"Well, if you drink enough beer along with your dinner it tends to just slide right out come morning." I killed. There was an applause break. Glad we got that out of the way, so I could make that awesome joke which was actually a true strategy I was employing, but it got a huge laugh, so I'll call it a joke. Glad we got that out of the way, so we could get to the real business of promoting me.

"And you're losing weight?!"

Ok. still pizza diet discussion. Fine. Though I was getting hungry with all this pizza talk.

"Yeah I'm losing weight! It's the best diet ever. I recommend it to anyone looking to be happy, lose weight and save money and time on food." Raucous laughter again.

"Amazing."

The laughter slowed down and then there was a beat of silence.

"Keep it up!"

And the door opened, and everyone left.

I went to the Little Caesars in Beverly Hills to drown my sorrows, but it had closed down. I ended up going to a cash only chicken-themed pizza spot by my old apartment that was takeaway only. I ate it in my car. I savored every bite. Stayed there a bit longer than I probably should have. Was in no hurry to get back to work.

8. "PARMESAN: THE STINKY CHEESE."

I was training for my first marathon and the run that day called for five miles. It was my first training cycle, so I had yet to fully appreciate running early in the morning and having a whole day afterwards with no workout hanging over my head. I slept in, had brunch, took a nap, had lunch and a soda, then watched tv for a couple hours before getting my stuff together about an hour before dark. A five-mile run took me about fifty minutes at the time and my girlfriend - now my wife, was going to make dinner while I was out, gnocchi.

I did my normal five-mile route. About two miles in I started to have a side stitch on my right side. Over the next mile the pain spread across my stomach quickly, from the right ascending, through the transverse, into the left descending colon. It was gurgling and bubbling in the way only a fart does, so when it finally got to the ole back door I slowly let it squeeze out while running. Over the next mile I let two or three more out until I got to the bottom of the well, and it was more than air. I caught it just in time, but every step further saw the little bubble behind whatever terror lurked at the gate shake up like a soda can.

I was almost exactly one mile from home. In ten minutes, I could run one mile. I take about a hundred and eighty steps per minute, so once I discovered the pressurized poo had reached the end of the line I had about eighteen hundred opportunities for catastrophe, each of which was closer to happening than the last. Each of which increased the amount of force, effort and concentration I needed to employ to keep that round in the chamber.

I made it back to my apartment, but my GPS said four point nine miles. I was supposed to run five miles but cut a corner due to a red light. I was about a tenth of a mile short. I ran past my apartment until I reached the five-mile mark. Once I hit it I stopped running immediately and started walking the block or two back to my apartment. I had to cross a street at a stop sign that was often blown through by impatient West LA drivers, so when I saw a car blasting down the street, I waited on the curb to see if I would be safe to cross, as jumping out of the way of a two thousand-pound BMW would surely be my undoing. Unfortunately, it stopped, and the driver motioned for me to cross.

I was nicer, though, and waved her to go ahead. She would not take no for an answer and waited. I took three steps into the crosswalk when another wave hit. The move is to stop, clench and squeeze the butt-cheeks, or in the event of DEFCON number two, drop to a knee and sit on the heel of your shoe letting your weight and the hard rubber heel of your shoe combine forces to beat the pressure. I was in a crosswalk, though and someone was waiting, so I hesitated. I hesitated and shit my pants right there in that crosswalk in front of that BMW. I kept walking, and whether they saw it or not, I'll never know. I got to the other side with an empty gut and full shorts and a need for rapid decisive action. I couldn't just go upstairs. My girlfriend was there. We had just moved in with each other a few months before and even if we hadn't, we were (and still are) very many years away from teaming up to solve a pant-shitting conundrum.

I was next door to our apartment complex. My plan was to get behind our dumpster, remove my shoes, which were by now absorbing the wateriest parts of my accident, take off my shorts and underwear, throw away the underwear, clean off with my shirt, throw that away and then show up to my apartment with no shirt and no shoes, say I puked and had to throw them both away, jump in the shower before dinner and never have to explain any of it. That plan worked, for the most part. The shoes were new, though and my wife is cheap. She wasn't afraid of a little bit of puke. She talked me into getting them out of the dumpster and cleaning them.

I showered, put on clean clothes and went into recovery mode. I had left a mess next to the dumpster which was also in the parking lot, so if I was going to be rooting around near the dumpster, I risked catching the blame for it. I filled a bucket with water and took the long way to the parking area to avoid running into neighbors. Somehow, I saw a lady from another unit and she said something to me, but I was in tunnel mode and I can't even tell you if I responded with words or a grunt or anything at all. All I can tell you is that I had a bucket of water to dump on a pile of my own doodie that flopped out of my underwear as I took it off to throw away after pooping my pants as a full grown up so I could rescue my doodie filled shoes because the lie I told my wife made it unreasonable to not salvage them.

I put them in the bucket and brought them back upstairs, filled the bucket with hot soapy water and soaked my shoes in it on the patio. I had gotten away with it. I washed my hands and sat down for dinner. The gnocchi was drenched in marinara sauce and covered in the tell-tale heart, parmesan cheese. Every time the breeze was right I'd catch a whiff of the cheese and think for half a second, that I had missed a bit in the shower, or that my shoes -- soaking on the porch, would betray me somehow. The guilt, however, would never overcome me and I would run the San Francisco marathon in those shoes a few months after they were soaked in my own shit.

9. "DIVISION OF LABOR."

Firehouse pizza was owned by the old dude with the Ugg boots and the Salem cigarettes. The bulk of the staff were his grandkids and they were all in high school. They worked the line - making the food and taking orders and running it and bussing, and the drivers would take deliveries and wash the dishes. None of the kids were old enough to be a driver, so that left a bunch of non-family members as drivers. Washing the dishes was one of the things I didn't expect about the job. It taught me a lot about eating at restaurants -- the plates probably aren't as clean as you think, and about washing dishes at home - beyond getting all the stuff off them they can only get so clean. I learned that a sink full of hot water will take cheese off a plate or a lasagna pan with no scrubbing at all - pretty much anything will fall off a plate if the water is hot enough and there's soap in it. I also learned how much being tall made stooping over a sink incredibly painful for my lower back. The dishwashing was just busy work most of the shift and then a big final sprint at the end of the night. Hovering over a steamy sink in a cramped kitchen with ten other people surrounding an enormous six-hundred-degree block of stone and steel was as close to a workout as I got at the time and just as sweaty.

Most of the shift was spent staring at a map and memorizing directions. This was before smartphones, and there was a giant map that we would have to plan our routes on by hand - sometimes four stops at a time. I also spent a lot of time driving, and smoking cigarettes. I smoked a cigarette on the way to and from every delivery which expanded my habit to well over a pack a day. The cash was so good, though. My take home pay from 5 shifts a week in a pizza shop was not eclipsed by my real jobby need a degree job until four years after college.

The grand kids were alright to work with. They and their high school friends all worked with us older drivers and weren't intimidated at all. I would call us friends but that would be super weird. We never hung out. They never even asked me to buy them beer or anything. I never thought much of that until right now and suddenly I am kind of offended. I always thought they thought I was cool, but I guess they had a cooler booze connect or liked talking to bums or another, younger driver bought it for them. I guess we would've been friends if we were the same age. They were all metalheads, and I liked metal. They liked pizza, and I loved pizza. We all lived in the same town. What else would you need to be friends except be the same age?

The drivers were all roughly the same age as I was. When I first started three of my closest friends at the time were also drivers, which is how I got the job. They didn't take their work very seriously and within three months they'd all been trimmed to one shift per week and quit. It was a huge bummer at first, but once my friends left I started being friendlier with the rest of the staff and liking the gig a whole lot better, which is saying a lot because the gig involved essentially an unlimited supply of pizza and pizza related goods like calzones, pasta and anything I could invent with the resources at my disposal.

My first item was pepperoni fried chicken. I took a bunch of pepperonis and dropped it in a hot skillet. Once the fat from it had been rendered, I pulled those little crispy things out and set them aside to snack on later, then dropped in some pre-cooked chicken strips to cook in the hot oil. Once the chicken was heated up in the pepperoni oil I would put it on a sub roll, top it with the crispy pepperoni slices and then go absolutely insane on it. Every time I ate that thing was like my first time eating anything. It was such a good sandwich that it almost made up for the fact that it wasn't a pizza. After a while I figured that anything worth heating up in a skillet was worth heating up in rendered pepperoni fat and the lasagna and spaghetti I made, along with the cheese spread where you just mix the pepperoni oil and parmesan cheese, were staples in my diet when I wanted a salty snack.

Another favorite of mine was pizza with pasta sauce. Not exactly original, but everyone else was stuck in their own baby brains only making what was on the menu and I was casting my worldly gaze internally and absolutely feasting. Calzone with no cheese but a ton of BBQ sauce and chicken and pineapple? I ate that. I called it a Polynesian pizza pocket which may or may not have been racist, I still don't know. There was a deep fryer in the back as well - a small capacity one that could get through about a half dozen chicken wings at a time. I never did anything with it. I don't find fried foods that interesting. I don't know why. I did put a bunch of cashews into a food processor and make cashew butter which I then put on a pizza crust that I cooked with nothing on it once. That was too much trouble and didn't slow down the ulcerative colitis flare I was having at the time as I had hoped, though, so I only did it once.

Between delivering the food, washing the dishes and making food - which is alarming in hindsight as I did not and still do not have a food handler's certificate, which is apparently a prerequisite for working in a kitchen, I got to know the other drivers pretty well. The few who worked there for any length of time. On Fridays, I worked with one of the older nephews of the owner. He the weekday afternoon driver and would need help on Fridays for the big Friday lunch rush, so I would roll in around eleven and work until the beginning of the dinner rush when another swing driver would roll in and help the two night drivers. Every now and again I would catch a double and work from eleven to eleven if a night driver didn't show up and the night swing driver couldn't cover or whatever. Those days I would leave with about three hundred dollars cash plus two days' worth of time thanks to the long shift and three free meals (one when I showed up, one at dinner break and one to take home), and whatever wine I could sneak into my soda cup. Huge. Those days were rare though, happening only about once a month.

The nephew was a townie, Riverside born and raised. He had played baseball in college before he dropped out. His head was shaved but he had a long goatee. We talked a lot about baseball and facial hair care but never anything of substance. The owners were often gone during the morning shifts as he was family and could be trusted and they had to go get their kids to and from school and practices and manage the other shop and whatever it is that grownups do during the day. Nothing weird ever happened with that guy though. He eventually left to go work at a train company. I only mention him because we spent a lot of time together - like thirty Fridays in a row and never connected at all. I've had more in common with most of my cab drivers than I did with this person. And yes, he used conditioner for his goatee.

Dewey started the same time as me. His name wasn't actually Dewey, but we called him that because he looked like that kid Dewey from "Malcolm in the Middle." His nickname was so prevalent that the owners began putting him on the schedule as "Dewey," and then his real name in parenthesis which I don't remember but I know it was something hella white and a bit trashy like Jake or Ricky. He was a spaz. Just too much energy and no control at all. Not a townie from riverside but a townie for sure. Townies always have batshit insane lives and he was no different. He was from Arizona but had to leave because he stole some tools from his dad and got kicked out of his house and told him he was going to kill him. He was going to the local community college, lived with his drug dealer in exchange for keeping the house clean, and delivered pizzas in his grandmother's old car from which he refused to remove the fuchsia hibiscus flower seat covers.

He would always come back to the shop and describe the people he just delivered pizzas to, but only if they were hot chicks. He also seemed to constantly be hooking up with or exchanging phone numbers with or delivering to them in various states of undress. Stories which I hated to hear because yuck, but also because I knew they were outright lies. I'm sure he just wanted us to like him but every time he left we would joke about what dumb story he was going to tell next. I have no clue what happened to him. I don't remember if he stopped working there before I left or the other way around. The last memory I have of him is me being drunk at his house with a couple of my friends and scoring brown cocaine from his roommate / landlord but getting a good enough deal where we didn't care but then our feet sweat so we never bought from Tony again. Tony wasn't his name but when we called we were supposed to ask if Tony was around because Tony was the code name for cocaine because Scarface Tony Montana.

Another driver was the son of the night manager. Would you be surprised to know that he was a townie? His townie cred came on his last day when he discovered that he was implicated in some type of crime and there was a warrant out for his arrest, so his dad told him to drive the fuck to Colorado and he did. He just left work because he was wanted for a fucking crime and never came back.

The last two, and the two I spent the most time with were hilarious, but also townies. They liked the Kottonmouth Kings and they tucked their ears into their hats which didn't have any bend to the bill, leaving a weird gap that could either be filled with ears or push them out. Normal guys would bend their bill and avoid the situation, but the style for townies at the time was flat brims and tucked in ears. They both somehow had southern type accents despite being born and raised in California and they both worked the day shift at Domino's pizza in town. They were really scared of accidentally touching hands under water if both washing dishes at the same time. They both had the same group of friends who they had known since elementary school. They lived with each other and bickered like it. They also both had a wicked crush on the front desk girl who was studying to be a cosmetician.

Once after work I agreed to go with them to an Indian casino. It was a bit of a drive but we all decided to carpool. Somehow, we ended up in a fifteen-year-old two door Honda civic. Though I was the tallest of the three by at least six inches I chose the back seat, as being scrunched was preferable to having to sit up front with a kid who I hardly knew and barely liked. They kept the music low and we chit chatted on the way to the interstate, discussing mostly the very recent drunk driving death of a friend of theirs which they were still processing. They were really affected by it. All of the things I used to think about them came into question. These were normal men who didn't choose where to be born and though they were too scared or comfortable to leave, that didn't make them any less human. I felt sorry for them, though I had yet to lose any friends, I could empathize with how they must feel at that time, how life seemed so fragile and impermanent and how they would struggle for the rest of their lives at the loss they suffered before they knew what it meant to lose.

Then we got to the freeway and they pulled out a blunt and cranked the Kottonmouth Kings through the aftermarket sound system before I could question the wisdom behind mourning a friend -- who died driving drunk, by driving high. The best I could muster was to refuse to smoke with them but then the freeway noise became too much and up went the windows, so I had no choice but to get high. Thirty minutes later we were at the casino. I was pretty high; just high enough to be uncomfortable around the civilians that weren't high in the casino, but the other two were straight up dinosaur high.

Dinosaur high happens to everyone if you smoke enough. It's clear to everyone besides you that you are high as fuck. You basically turn into a dinosaur. Your eyes bulge. Your head leans forward and pulls you off balance. Your elbows dig into your ribs and your palms face in, fingers spread and claw like as your subconscious reptilian brain is trying to keep you from falling on your face with every step you prance toward wherever you think you need to go at the time which is usually to indulge some base desire like food or sleep or water. Or poker, as was the case on this night.

The poker room was full. Or we were too high to figure out the subtle complexities of wait lists, table changes and the other confusing bits of casino poker. Whichever it was, somehow the prevailing wisdom was that we needed to go to another casino forty-five minutes away. Back in the car, another blunt and hot box journey and we were there, though by this time we were cooked and sat for only a couple hours before calling it a night. I never hung out with them again outside of work.

10. "UNSAFE VS UNCOMFORTABLE."

The best pizza I've ever had was cooked in a microwave. In March of 2015, a mere four months before The Great Pizza Experiment began, I went to Yosemite National Park. It was a low snow year, so we figured that early in the season we could get pretty far into the backcountry. We drove up early on a Wednesday and walked into the visitor's center to get our permit. The ranger wasn't sure how deep the snow was and where but gave us a permit and wished us luck.

We ate chicken strips and french fries and pulled out a map to plot our course. Eating lunch before a backpacking trip never bodes well for big miles, but it was just after daylight saving time and our first camp was only a half day away, so we were okay spending a little time. The walk was beautiful. For those who have never been to Yosemite National Park, it's a big fucking deal for a reason and better writers than me have spent entire careers trying to convey the magnitude to which being in this green splotch on the map will simultaneously humble you beneath its unimaginable grandeur, while in so doing make you soar.

The trail we were taking on - The Mist Trail runs about three and a half miles from The Happy Isles trailhead to the top of Nevada Fall. It is so heavily trafficked that the granite trail from it to our final destination for the night has been ground to beach sand by all the rubber boot steps over the hundred years it's been walked. It's such a busy trail that the trash on top sustains an entire population of yellow jackets, mice, and snakes. It is the portal from the world-famous Yosemite Valley to the world-famous high sierra backcountry. It is so busy they built bathrooms up there, so people would stop leaving their poops out. So, when we got to the top about an hour before sunset and it was empty we were struck dumb. I have never and probably won't ever meet a person who's been alone on top of Nevada Fall and I became one. We didn't want to breathe for fear of spoiling the place's perfection. We only left to avoid hiking the last mile to camp in the dark.

We camped the first night in Little Yosemite Valley - a mini version of the Yosemite Valley you've undoubtedly seen in pictures. It was there, that first night between the fire and the tent when I caught a breeze and was cold. Not chilly, but actually cold. The base layer shirt I bought was barely long enough to cover my abnormally long and pudgy torso and the running tights I was using as base layer pants seemed to shed heat instead of trapping it. I'd be fine, though, my sleeping bag was rated to thirty degrees which was about the overnight low, and in case it wasn't I bought a little insert which was supposed to add a few degrees, so I was confident that I'd be ok no matter how cold it got, which I was that night.

The next day we got our typical city-start (wake up with the sun, casually eat breakfast, clean up camp and be walking by nine-am). Our goal was the sunrise lakes via the John Muir Trail, but with a bonus spur to Cloud's rest and back. Within an hour the trail was beneath snow. It started ankle deep and breaking through was just a bit of an energy suck, but as we climbed higher and higher the snow got deeper and deeper. By the time we stopped for lunch we were just following a river under the snow by ear. There were no other tracks out there. We were the first ones up for the season. When we stopped for lunch I complained a little. I was worried about post-holing and breaking my leg. The snow was only knee deep at the time, so I was being a baby, but my friend - a former wilderness guide, gave me a little pep talk. It was very little. "You're uncomfortable, you are not unsafe."

That really made it better. We continued on past lunch. Met up with a solo Italian hiker who was coming from the direction we were going who told us it was unpassable ahead without snowshoes or skis. We decided we wanted to go see for ourselves, as hikers have the tendency to lie to other hikers about things as a way of asserting their outdoor dominance. It happens all the time and to everyone. It's the one thing I hate about hiking and backpacking, hikers' advice.

It can be as simple as wrong mileage, or wrong time estimates which can be explained away as just not being aware, so fine. As late-starters, my wife and I get the ole "you're not gonna make it before dark," pretty much any time we ever stop and chat with hikers - and the only time we've ever hiked in the dark is to catch the sunrise. I've even had hikers stop me and warn me about my choice of footwear. Yes, a septuagenarian with a BMI in the 30's had the nerve to stop me on my way back to camp from half-dome to tell me my shoes were all wrong. Ugh. Hikers. Shut up. And stop playing music on the trail. It's disgusting.

In this situation, however, the Italian was right. Immediately after we passed him we crossed a snow bridge over a stream and lost the trail for good. Our friend split up to go look for the trail and the stream was too loud to find each other quickly. Once we regrouped we tried to gain the pass but near the top the snow was hip deep and we all agreed continuing on would be foolish as there wasn't even a clear spot in which to camp, so we turned around and backtracked. We made camp at around nine thousand feet in a clearing and melted snow to drink. It was a gorgeous campsite and our fire that night was tiny but hot. My wife lost a sock trying to dry it too close to the fire and despite my dry clothing I was unable to get truly warm.

Again, I caught a serious chill on the way from the fire to the tent. This was the night I discovered that a sleeping bag doesn't work to its rating if you can't zip it up, which I couldn't because I'm a bigger man. Not fat, necessarily, but not thin, and with broad shoulders, a barrel chest, a gut and gangly gorilla arms there was just too much to zip into the bag. Plus, I was still foolishly wearing the damn tights that made me cold. I woke up every hour, did some sleeping bag sit ups to warm up and then was able to fall asleep again. The night felt like it was taking forever and what made it worse is that I had to pee but didn't want to get out of my bag to do it, so it made it just that much colder and more uncomfortable because holding in pee makes you cold.

The next day we hiked to a high alpine lake and had it all to ourselves the same way we had Nevada Falls to ourselves two nights before. The trails we were walking are hiker superhighways. The places we were stopping are on postcards. We were undisturbed, except for the Italian, for fifty hours in a row and if it takes a couple nights shivering and worried a little bit about hypothermia, that's fine. It's not fine, it's stupid and when I got home I would buy better gear, but you get my point.

We camped above the lake to get away from the mosquitos on the shore. This night was only noteworthy because I had to pee so bad that I got out of my tent to do it, and to my horror, the dew on the rainfly had frozen in strips that caught the blue light of the waxing moon and I felt like I was under water. After I peed I slept hard and woke up well after sunrise. We got moving and fifteen miles later we were back to the car. It was too late to drive home though. We had one more night to sleep out.

I had run out of water about a mile before we got to camp. It was a long day, so I didn't think much of it until I unpacked my pack and discovered my sleeping bag was soaked from a leak in my hydration bladder. I had been cold all week with a dry bag, I was horrified to have to sleep in a wet one. We laid it out on the table and I repeated my friend's mantra in my head as anxiety boiled quickly to the surface. I was not unsafe, I was just uncomfortable.

We took a bus to the pizza place in Yosemite Valley - Declan's attic or something. But we were horrified to discover it was closed for the season. A wet sleeping bag and the pizza I'd been looking forward to all day was closed. Not unsafe, uncomfortable. But as I shook the locked doors of the pizza place in hopes it would change the reality, we hatched a backup plan. A cafeteria in a hotel who's name I don't remember and has since changed when the concessionaire who ran it for the parks service took their trademarks after being replaced was open year-round and they had "everything."

It was just around the corner. We walked in and I quickly scanned the room. No pizza station but there was a freezer. Freezers are hope. Anything can be in a freezer, and this place had everything. Including pizza? I ripped the fogged-up door open and scanned the packaging. This was the ice cream freezer! Next door, more fog but I opened it just as quickly. Pizza! I gave it to a man in an apron and a beard net. While he microwaved it for me, I went and grabbed as many single beer bottles as I could carry - cafeterias only sell singles, apparently. I paid and got a table.

By the time my personal pizza was done I had already drank a beer and I was feeling it pretty good. We decided not to stop for lunch in order to get back to the valley with enough time to eat and get back to camp before sundown, so I hadn't eaten lunch. I had hiked fifteen miles since my last meal and had only eaten dehydrated chicken and rice and canned chicken salad for the past four days. When they say hunger is the best sauce, they make no mention of exhaustion, anxiety, light drunkenness and lack of variety which are incredible sauces all on their own but in concert they made for the best frozen pizza I've ever had in my life.

I don't remember the brand of pizza, but it was about four inches across and deep dish. Four stubby pre-cut slices rejoined with bubbly blistery white cheese floating atop the sauce. There was a salty crust of cheese around the edge that had fried in its own oil as it sweat out in the microwave and if you got too greedy it would snap off on the way to your mouth. The bottom was crispy, too, for a microwave pizza and it wasn't because it was burnt through like some of those thinner microwave pies. I ate the pizza in bullet time. Like a movie, every time the pie crossed my lips the din of the room warped down and the lights went off and my eyes slid shut as I savored every chew of every bite. When I swallowed it was like I had time traveled a very short distance into the future. It was pure glory. It was neither unsafe nor uncomfortable.

After dinner, we bought a sixer at the store and grabbed some sweatpants from my car. I was fully prepared to get drunk enough to sleep wet - I'd done it before when I mixed alcohol and hydrocodone in college, pissed my bed but was too stoned and drunk to care so I just slept through it, so I was confident I would be ok. When we got back to the campsite by some pizza induced karmic miracle my sleeping bag was dry. I breathed a deep sigh of relief and got drunk in celebration. I slept hard again only waking to pee once before waking with the sun and joining a neighboring campsite's morning fire to hear about the bear that sniffed my buddy's face as he "cowboy camped," (slept out in a sleeping bag on the ground instead of in a tent, bivy sack or hammock), and enjoyed the rest of the morning in what very well may turn out to be the center of the universe before driving home in traffic, and jumping in the pool instead of showering.

11. "BUZZ."

I woke up on the first day of the third week of The Great Pizza Experiment down almost seven pounds. I shot out of bed. There was no reason to hit snooze. The faster I got up the faster I could get ready and go to work and work out and then do the one thing I wanted to spend the rest of my life doing: eating pizza.

The singular focus provided by having no food decisions to make allowed my brain to work at full speed. For example: I invented a combination pool cover and trampoline that will save lives, turn backyards into playgrounds and make me a billionaire as soon as Mark Cuban reads this book (get at me Mark). As this was during deflategate I developed a strategy for the NFL to defeat Tom Brady - hire Eli Manning as their attorney. I tweeted it at them a couple times, but they never responded.

My finest achievements, however, per normal, were pizza related. Since all I was eating was pizza and still logging forty miles a week I needed some portable za to eat while running. It's still in the pre-prototype phase but I think it's the next big thing for endurance sports after energy bars, gels, energy waffles, fruit, carbohydrate drinks, electrolyte drinks, jelly beans, boiled potatoes and salt, pretzels, peanut butter sandwiches, oatmeal, spam musubi, and Oreos.

On the same road but not necessarily sports related, I came up with the idea of popcorn pizza. Not popcorn shrimp on pizza. Shrimp is weird, especially pizza shop shrimp. I don't want it anywhere near my pizza. Not popcorn chicken on a pizza, either, although I would totally fuck with that. Popcorn pizza is little baby pizzas that are battered and fried. Maybe they could be called pizza nuggets or pizza tenders. Whatever they're called, once I get around to making a ton of them, they're going to be way popular.

The third week was also the week where everyone I knew started getting super involved with the bet and expressing a rooting interest. People would send me stuff. Some of it was cool like, "Hey check out this pizza restaurant that has a shrine to Frank Sinatra in it," or "Check out this pizza restaurant in your neighborhood that I've had and is great." Some of the stuff people shared was dumb as fuck though. They meant well so I was always grateful but who wants a cake that's covered in fondant in order to look like a pizza? Get that counterfeit pizza out of here! Fondant tastes like shit and ever since Cakeboss came around it's everywhere and it's objectively disgusting so stop pretending it isn't and stop covering cakes in it. If I want cake I make a cake. If I want pizza I make a pizza. Not everything has to be everything else! Like my attorney said, "as a student of Boytosian exploits, this may take the cake. But only if that cake is made of cheese bread and meat!" Cheese and meat, not fondant!

I wrote my first book while I was conducting the great pizza experiment. It only took me one night. The book was called "The Real Secret" and it was one page long and that page said, "eat pizza and nothing else." My attorney said, "do not publish this book it is a bad book and also probably stealing some juice from 'the secret' so they'll probably sue you and I'm not actually a real lawyer I'm just your golfing buddy," so I followed his advice. But if the secret people are looking for a sequel get at me.

The dumbest shit I heard during The Great Pizza Experiment was about how unhealthy it was. None of my friends are nutritionists, but somehow a bunch of them were able to read, understand and compare my diet with a study that was going around at the time. The study was basically people eating six thousand calories a day and lying in bed. I think I received this article a half dozen times in a week. I didn't engage in debate because people are touchy about their diets and the pizza movement didn't need me besmirching its good name. However, the diet I was on was roughly one fourth of the calories and averaged twelve workouts per week. I'll say again:

there is a world of difference between eating only pizza and eating too much pizza.

Eating only pizza is not on its own an unhealthy thing to do. Thanks to my ulcerative colitis I have copious amounts of blood work to look back on. While eating nothing but pizza for the duration of The Great Pizza Experiment my HDL cholesterol went up, and my LDL went down. My triglycerides were unaffected, my liver function panels revealed no relevant changes, my folate deficiency was unchanged, and the rest of my bloodwork was normal. Am I saying an all pizza diet would do the same for you? No. I am a genetic freak. They say you can't outrun a bad diet and since my weight got closer to healthy non-overweight and my bloodwork was unharmed and even improved, the only conclusion is that eating only pizza is not a bad diet for me.

Another popular "Hey Greg look at this lol," was the pizza pocket. During the great pizza experiment, I received a link to this product no less than twenty times and since completing the experiment another twenty at least. Imagine if you will, a nerdy necklace that you would wear to a trade show or work conference, a clear plastic pouch in which you display your name tag or badge or credentials or whatever. If you've been to these conferences or anything like them, you know that these are very embarrassing things to wear and once you are issued one, you hide them in your breast pocket and only take it out if security hassles you, or if you need a stamp for some free shit.

Now imagine that as a triangle that can hold one slice of pizza. Again, everyone who shared it was so excited that I didn't want to yuck their yum with a trolley shitpost because I was thankful they were thinking of me and I always will be, but I have some notes for the product creator. First, it carries a weird size slice. It's not adjustable at all. Do you have one for every style of pizza? What if I have a Sicilian slice that needs to come with me? New York style? What about one of those super skinny slices from round table? Inadequate! Second, one slice? Am I a bird? Who needs just one slice so bad that they're putting it on a nerdy ass necklace and leaving the house with it? Not me. Third and finally, there was no purchase link. It was just a novelty item that wasn't actually for sale. Which was a major bummer because I would've bought one for sure. Not because I need it, but because I must have it.

Wednesday of this week I started craving dessert pizza. As luck would have it, the internet is full of wonderful dessert pizza recipes, so I had a lot to choose from once I started looking. I made one for the next three nights and ate the whole thing every time. There was little doubt that dessert pizza was pizza. Of course, it is. But why? Well what is pizza? It's dough, sauce and toppings all cooked at the same time. That's what every pizza is with few exceptions. At the time of print I can think of one exception: french bread pizza. Boboli is rarely pizza because the crust is already fully cooked. What do you call a fully cooked crust that you add toppings to and then cook? A grilled cheese. No offense Boboli but come on. You've had Boboli.

Saturdays during The Great Pizza Experiment were the best. Usually we'd go rock climbing, grab food and bring it to a brewery and hang hard. The Saturday of the third week, though, we were out of town and the best brewery around was Pizza Port. If that sounds pizza-y it's because it's a pizza restaurant as well. They do sandwiches too. But pizza does strange things to people. A week earlier, right before falling asleep, my girlfriend asked if we could have one cheat day a week. I said she could, but I would stick to the bet as agreed upon. On this Saturday, the day after her weekly cheat day, menu in hand, she made the hard choice.

She chose pizza.

She forfeited the pizza vs sandwich bet by choosing pizza. Not chicken and vegetables or a salad or soup or sushi or Chinese food or anything aside from the one true enemy to the sandwich diet: pizza. That's the incredible pull that pizza has. It can convert its biggest skeptic to completely sell out and lose everything sacred to them to eat it. Dangerous parallels aside, the pizza power is incredible. She quit. She lost. Sandwiches were demonstrably less appealing than pizza on a meal to meal, week to week and month to month basis.

My girlfriend had to give me five dollars comment on the original debate comment threat, and make a new post declaring me the victor and pizza the superior food. She did. It's tough to say which was more excruciating for her, admitting defeat, announcing defeat, or losing five dollars. She is so cheap. There's not even a punchline for that. She is just a very cheap human. It's such a part of her personality that she does this little cute bird noise (because her name is Robin) and it's just a chirp but instead of actually chirping it's "cheap cheap!" it's cute but she's also very cheap and proud of her cheapness so the five dollars was very likely the worst part of losing for her. I still have the five-dollar bill she turned over to me. I keep it in a box on my dresser next to the last dollar I was down to before having to give up and move back home. Both of those bills changed my life and I'll never spend either.

The comment thread exploded again. People asked if I was shocked that it lasted less than three weeks. I was not. I've had pizza before and sandwiches too and it was clear to me which would outlast which. I was shocked anyone would make the bet, but not shocked it was such a short affair. Also, I knew from previous experience that my girlfriend was made of jello. We did a week-long cookie diet - with special diet cookies, and she lasted less than a day. She did that cayenne pepper and lemon juice and maple syrup cleanse the year before we met and often joked that she didn't even finish the first day. Was I surprised? No, not at all.

I was surprised at the rallying of support for pizza in its moment of triumph. People were let down by the shortness of the bet. The first comment was telling, "Congratulations Greg, having a pizza to celebrate? #teampizza" I thought that was a good idea, and there were leftovers from lunch, so I crushed them and fell asleep a champion. I woke up the next morning emboldened. I knew that one pizza as a victory lap wouldn't be enough, and the internet agreed. The bet was done but The Great Pizza Experiment had just begun. It was me vs. time.

How long could I go? This was a once in a lifetime opportunity to truly live my dream with no judgement, no outside interference, no petty fights about all I wanted to eat was pizza and how boring that was. I was able to live my dream and have everyone behind me in full force in unanimous approval and support. That kind of shit only happens to young money and I see how fast it gets out of control. People wanted to talk to me, people invited me to lunch, people would check in with me and for no money at all! That last sentence sounds really sad, but it's only kind of sad. Some people go out of their way to connect with me on a regular basis, but not such a huge amount and not usually so enthusiastic.

Along with the success came the next challengers. They all reached out in their own way, privately, and said they thought my girlfriend was admirable in her effort but also likely not the best candidate to represent team sandwich. I think that was underselling the obvious superiority of pizza, and also kind of rude to my girlfriend. They were all very polite about it though, mostly because they were afraid of her. She is a certified badass with years of kickboxing training and over fifty NCAA rugby matches under her belt. I'm still scared of her to this day. But physical fear isn't willpower. They were right, and polite enough about it to keep me from snitching on them to my girlfriend. It's a real bet killer to invite a fresh challenger in while you're in the middle of something, though, but I was a true believer, so I gave them a chance. I told them all the same thing, "Eat nothing but sandwiches for a week and then call me," and to this day not even one of them has. Probably because they can't give up pizza.

After three weeks of The Great Pizza Experiment I was down 7.8 pounds total and I could shoot noisy stars out of my hands or whatever Jubilee's dumb power was. I don't even know where to start with that hot take. I don't like comic books, but I don't hate comic books or people who like comic books. I even used to watch the x-men cartoon on tv when I was a kid, so I don't hate the x-men. Her power sucked though, I think. Fight me.

12. "FIGHTS."

Please don't fight me. I am a tremendous coward. In my life, I've never been in a fight. I used to tell a story that took place at an In-n-Out Burger in which I punched a kid heroically for bad mouthing my girlfriend at the time, but that story is a lie. Just before my first senior year of college I was very nearly in a fight at the campus pizza place but was the odd man out, too far away, busy doing something else and also a coward so I merely watched. The summer before my second senior year I started a fight in the same pizza place, but my girlfriend at the time broke it up before it got beyond spitting on a person. Once during the great pizza experiment a wino almost got his ass kicked by my friend for threatening a female next to whom I was standing with sexual violence.

I can't think of any other close calls with regards to me and fights, and I don't know how I should feel about that. I know I feel proud because while others are at boring ass salad shops, I'm usually in the middle of a pizza place, which is awesome prima facie. I know I also feel scared that pizza makes me into a more quarrelsome individual, but then I run back the tape, on which I am a reputed coward and realize that pizza places are just the lowest common denominator as far as clientele, more so than anywhere else I spend time. This makes me feel relieved. The fact that I find so much disagreement in pizza places is likely everyone else's fault. There is never any actual violence, though. I escape as far ahead of the violence as possible, sometimes at a detriment to my social life. Luckily, sometimes I lack the foresight to escape before catastrophe, so I can experience it vicariously through the vertebrates I spend time with.

Before my first senior year in college, I had just turned 21 and was able to drink legally in California. I had a bit of money on account of my sweet job that provided for my room and board in addition to a small monthly stipend which I would have drank in two weeks, easily were it not for one pesky rule: since the apartment they gave me was in the residence halls I could not consume or possess alcohol in it. For all of my faults and fuckups, this is a rule I obeyed remarkably strictly, only slipping up once. It technically wasn't even my fault since I was carrying a backpack in which a friend had stored some faderade - a lovely mix of clear liquor and Gatorade. I blacked out, Irish goodbye'd everyone, puked in my kitchen sink, slept in my empty bathtub and didn't discover the alcohol until I woke up dehydrated and thirsty. I dug through the backpack, found the Gatorade bottle and guzzled it before the taste of the gin hit me and I barfed it all back up.

Not being able to drink at home meant that I needed friends who could and would keep up with my pace and endurance, as well as friends that didn't mind always drinking at their place. Failing that, I needed to spend a ton of time in bars. I wore out my welcome pretty quickly, and to preserve our friendships I think we decided bars were best. It was Riverside, California in the early twenty-aughts, we could afford to throw down at a bar when 60 oz. pitchers went for five bucks, and someone cleaned up after you.

As it happened, the closest bar to campus was also primarily a pizza restaurant. I say restaurant because I want to seem less sad. It was a bar that served pizza. It had a pool table, a pop-a-shot, a big screen tv and a huge outdoor patio. It was a five-minute walk from most of my classes and my apartment, near enough the commuter student parking lots and close to the off-campus apartments at which my friends all lived. The pizza was good, too: whole milk mozzarella, canned sauce but with some extra additions to temper the sweetness and the tin-ness out of it, hand tossed crust, they used flour to keep it from sticking instead of corn meal and they used a stone, not a conveyor belt. Did I mention $5 pitchers? This place was called "The Getaway Cafe," and I loved it.

The week before school starts every year the school puts on a block party. There's a concert, carnival activities, the fraternities and sororities set up for recruitment and everyone just has a good ole time. Some people choose to use this event as an excuse to over-consume alcohol and make poor decisions. I am one of those people. I also hung out with most of the rest of those people.

We showed up drunk as a result of a healthy pre-party at our friends' apartment. Four of them had been living together since freshman year and their apartment became our surrogate neutral ground for pre-festivity festivities. I think I funneled a bottle of yellowtail shiraz and then did some shots. We all shotgunned beers and smoked cool cigarettes like lucky strikes, because Marlboro was too mainstream, or they were on sale I can't remember which. Since I worked on campus I tried to keep my wits about me, a practice that somehow included funneling wine, but it made sense at the time, and we eventually ventured out to the block party.

That part of every western film when the town is just going about its business and the thunder of hooves in the distance gives everyone a sense of looming danger and then it's revealed it's the bad guys riding in, is exactly how I would categorize us rounding the corner on campus and appearing to the normal folks at the block party. We were not there to raise hell, just have fun, but we looked drunk, unpredictable and maybe a little bit dirty and dangerous. It was hot. The sun was going down. We were separated from each other instantly in the huge crowd and somehow, we met up on the other side of it a quarter mile away, except for one of us.

This was a problem, of course, but we thought it was hilarious that the drunkest one out of all of us – historically and presently – was missing and wrecked in a crowd of decent humans. We laughed but we all set back into the crowd immediately on a rescue mission. Not to rescue him from it but to rescue it from him. We echo located him by following the sound of his booming laugh and found him behind a dumpster. He was unlocking the wheels of the dumpster. Then he was pushing the dumpster. And the laughing. A lot of laughing. And then he was pushing the dumpster somehow harder than the four of us could resist. And then he was running.

Into the street. Like Frogger. If cars slammed on their brakes and honked at Frogger while Frogger ran past them screaming "fuck you!" He made it across and into The Getaway unscathed but that didn't mean his problems were over. We needed backup.

His girlfriend was called. She was on her way. All we had to do was keep him inside until she could get there. So, we ordered pizza and way too much beer while we waited. The place was crowded but we snagged a table and began to hold court. Eventually we moved outside to have a cigarette. As the patio was full we stood very near to the street that was the main avenue to and from the block party that was still raging. A fraternity brother of one of my friends approached and asked to use one of their cell phones. It worked out to there being six of us and six of them, but I was standing back on the patio because I couldn't drink my beer on the street, and numbers didn't matter because these guys were brothers or whatever.

Suddenly the frat bro started screaming and one of my friends hit him in the face and it was on. There was a fight - my friends, punching, clenching, parrying, pushing, running, dodging and kicking. I couldn't believe what was happening. "A fight," I thought. "We were just having fun like three seconds ago and now they're rolling in the street!" I chugged my beer, tossed my cigarette down. "We're going to have to run away as soon as this settles down. There's still half a pizza left inside!" I ran inside, wrapped the leftover pizza in a bunch of napkins, finished a random beer on the table, tucked the pizza under my arm like a football and ran back outside.

It had just ended. Everyone was ok, but still drunk and panicking. We hurried back through the bar to the back door and through the parking lot and across another street where our drunk friend's girlfriend was just pulling up to acquire him. We all jumped in and screamed to "just fucking drive!" and she dutifully sped away with a bunch of drunk dudes freaking out in her car. It was fine. They didn't know I could've helped but didn't. They were all excitedly telling about their small corners of the brawl to ask me where I was the whole time. Had they asked I would've lied and said eating pizza and knowing me, they would've believed it.

That same patio of that same bar exactly one year later with those same friends and I'm sitting next to a girl I'm dating and there's only one other group at the bar and as they're leaving a guy starts yelling at her, how she's a bitch because she wouldn't give him her number after "all that fucking beer [he] gave [her]." Unwilling to let my lady's honor be called into question, and ignoring the fact that at $5 per pitcher he had spent $3 TOPS on her, I summarily dismissed the complainant's claim at deserving a phone number, disparaged his masculinity, jumped up and cocked my arm back to swing at the same time my friend (incidentally the same one that started the fight above) was spitting in this guy's face. My lady caught my wrist and said to stop, so I did.

That last one may not seem like an act of cowardice to the untrained eye, but it was. There was a fence between us, so I don't know what I was going to punch and I'm fairly certain that this made me act tougher than I was. That fence was basically a metaphor for the internet and I acted like a troll. This makes the only "fight," I haven't ducked out of or ran away from for non-coward reasons technically impossible and only did not proceed because I was henpecked out of it by a girl.

Fast forward ten long years of pizza peace, aside from a brief pizza delivery related mishap, and I'm standing in a Westwood village pizzeria with my improv team. I'm thirty and these kids range in age from twenty to twenty-five. Three still live at home, two who don't are still suckling at the teat of their parents and I, Greg Boytos, balding, with a mortgage and slightly overweight in six-year-old shoes am eating nothing but pizza on account of a bet I have with my wife. These poor kids get dragged along because this is the only place in Westwood I will eat pizza because the whole foods pizza is too expensive, the other places are either too far, aren't made properly are or straight up gross, and we all have to eat together because we have a comedy show in thirty minutes.

In walks a man carrying everything he owns in a backpack, and a wet paper shopping bag, haphazardly cradled in his arms like he's just been beamed back to earth from whatever alien spacecraft abducted him. The way the staff acknowledges him makes me feel like he's a regular. At first, he's jovial, greeting everyone in the place with a grin and pleasant, if boisterous hellos. At one point, he accidently knocks a cheese shaker to the ground and stoops to pick it up, tumbling everything cradled in his arms onto the floor. It's a lot of stuff and it's rolling around and I go out of my way to be nice to people who are so obviously in the midst of an attack of alcohol induced psychosis. I pick the stuff up for him.

He won't take the stuff back. I keep trying to hand it to him, but I am invisible to him. He's beginning to turn and there is a sudden edge on the nice things he's screaming about the pizza. He wants to order but he doesn't know what. Then he's overcome and wants to sing a song. He's got a decent voice, but he doesn't remember words and refuses to carry a tune. Soon he's just standing in front of the register chanting "fuck it fuck it fuck it fuck it" while my teammate tries to record him on his camera phone.

Then this guy's eyes shoot wide. I can see because I am the nearest one to him and I watch crazy people very carefully in case I have to describe them on twitter – a skill I learned from going to the urgent care at Kaiser Permanente. He puts his wet paper sack down, points an incredibly dirty finger at the only girl on our team – a bubbly blond in her early twenties, and screams that she's going to suck his fucking dick, which is the exact thing you should say if you ever want to turn an entire room of people against you. He makes a move towards her, and he has to pass me to do it.

He's not yelling anymore just doing that bum-grumble where he's just really agreeing with what he said – like an old prospector who smells gold, licking his lips and mumbling "oh yeah suck it good," and it's slow motion and my jaw is dropped, and I should say something or move into his way but he's fucking nuts. He's wearing a hospital bracelet so either he's just been let out of UCLA hospital or the VA hospital across the freeway. If it's the VA he's a vet and likely has been trained in combat and therefore doubly dangerous, and he stinks of cheap vodka, so his inhibitions are significantly lower, and pain tolerance higher. I'm holding his deodorant and toothpaste that I've picked up for him before this turned south and he's past me. I move to speak but can only huff out "hey, whoa," which has no effect on him.

My friend who was trying to record him slides his phone away, not getting good video at all when the youngest kid on my team, a model slash actor slash writer steps up, serious face as I've ever seen and holds his hand out as if to say "halt!" "What the fuck?!" is what he actually says and that's when a kid who worked at the pizza place, probably six feet four and three hundred pounds, gets in front of the crazy man and ushers him out the door without a fight.

The girl who was nearly assaulted thanked everyone out loud. We ordered and ate our pizza amid feverish apologies from the staff. Nobody said anything about how I could've blocked the way but didn't. Maybe nobody noticed except me. Maybe I'm too hard on myself because of my past cowardice. Maybe analysis paralysis is a thing that I have that causes me to think while others act. Maybe I live in constant fear. Only one thing is for sure, they do not give discounts when winos direct sexually aggressive language at members of your party.

13. "REGULARS."

As it was a local mainstay, an established locally owned business that had been around for a long while, Firehouse Pizza had some regulars. And if you can imagine the general weirdness of pizza shop regulars, plus the general weirdness of people who live in Riverside - who's municipal water district was headed by a member of the American Nazi party who ran unopposed every election, you could imagine there were some real noteworthy characters.

My first regular was Skateboard Dave. He was middle aged and lived remarkably close to the shop, but across a six-lane street. While it was technically walking distance, it was a death mission. Understanding this, he would order a small pepperoni and breadsticks with cheese for delivery, and we would just make a right, make a U-turn and make another right into his apartment complex. Dude was an excellent tipper despite the very little trouble it was to get his food to him. I think he was embarrassed because he could see the shop from his front door and so the tips were hush money, a payoff to escape judgment which was fine by me. I judged him more for being at home during regular work hours even though he was clearly an adult than for not wanting to cross a highway as stoned as he usually was.

To rectify this disconnect, I would make up stories about him. My brain needed to understand why a grown up with great taste in pizza and a bit of disposable income lived in a mediocre apartment in riverside that was decorated with skateboards - the dude had skateboard decks lining his wall like picket crown molding. My first theory was that he was a former pro skateboarder who had an injury and couldn't skate anymore, so he just sat around his apartment in his hometown and smoked pot and ate pizza. That held out for a couple months until I noticed the name on the skateboards wasn't the same. If he were a sponsored skater, he'd have his own custom boards with his name on them, not other people's!

Theory two: he was a skateboard designer. An artist who worked from home. That would explain the pot smell, the skateboards and the good tips. He couldn't create without chemical enhancement, proudly displayed the work he labored so hard to create and remembered what it was like as a young artist struggling to make ends meet with a service job while carving out time to hone his craft, so he liked to pay it forward to other tip-dependent people. Story two never got wrecked, but as a grownup myself, looking back I realize that story was too complex. Maybe the dude worked nights and liked skateboards. Maybe he worked from home - telecommuting as they call it. Perhaps he worked a job with floating or odd weekends. What if I stop making up origin stories about strangers and mind my own business?

And then there was Marcus from Central. One morning shift the phone rang. The boss was working the oven as the other driver was out on a delivery and the only other employee who wasn't in high school and could work the day-shift was on break, so I had to answer it. I wasn't trained how to answer the phones or anything but it's fucking easy to do if you've ordered as much pizza as I have. "Firehouse Pizza," I said, and waited for the other person to say what they wanted. They grunted. Not so much grunted as much as a groan. As if someone were bound and gagged and trying to call for help. Holy shit. Why would someone dial a pizza shop for help? Don't they know who works at places like these? Also, why push seven buttons instead of three for 911? Also, how do you dial but not just remove the rope/gag/tape?! "What?" I said. Panicking a little bit. The voice grunted again. "I can't hear you!" The panic subsided, and I started to get annoyed. It now sounded like the phone was in this person's mouth. Maybe they were super hungry! They grunted again. I was at a loss. "Hold on."

I briefed my boss on the situation. She smirked. "It's Marcus from Central."

"Marcus from Central?" I asked, not getting the joke. Boss lady just pointed to a pre-written ticket hanging on the bulletin board near the phone. It read "Marcus from Central," and had an order and an address. Two foot-long ham sandwiches NO OIL extra extra olives. Two two-liters of sprite. Cheesecake. I picked up the phone. "Marcus?" This time the grunt sounded like a happy confirmation. "Will you be having your usual?" Sounded again like an affirmative grunt. Even if it wasn't I don't know how we would change it up, so I made the food and took it to the address.

It was not a house or an apartment. There was a large lot, mostly dirt, near the airport. In the middle of this lot there was a strip mall that appeared to be under construction except there was no equipment around, so not under construction as much as unfinished. There was an asphalt parking lot with fresh lines but the driveway from the road to the parking lot was gravel. The building was wholly incongruous with itself. Three of the five store fronts had labels, but all of their windows were tinted. If there were a textbook for pizza delivery drivers on where you're going to be bound gagged and human trafficked, the graphic inset on the opposite page would be this parking lot. He was a regular, though, so either it was a remarkably long con or completely harmless.

When I pulled up a door opened revealing a slight, shirtless man in dirty jeans held up by a thick brown belt. He waved to get my attention, to signal that he, the only man in this parking lot was the one who had called. His jeans were so big he folded them over where the pleating would be on each side. He was tan and had close cropped hair. The whole situation had a remarkably feral vibe. He grunted out a "hey," or tried. It still sounded like he had a phone in his mouth. I nodded. He had a check, it was pre-approved by the boss lady. This guy had cache with the shop, so I treaded lightly, plus the check was for three dollars more than the tab which was a good tip considering how close the trip was.

I made polite small talk as I handed the food over. "Sorry I couldn't hear you on the phone, I listen to my music too loud," I said. It's a good tactic, blaming yourself is disarming and allows the person to whom you're attempting to ingratiate yourself to have the upper hand and show how honorable they can be by absolving you of your confessed crimes. He grinned when I said it and grunted some more at me. At this point I was in real trouble. I didn't hear a word, and this was small talk. There was a short time in which to respond but I hadn't a clue as to the direction to go as I hadn't understood a single syllable out of Marcus' mouth.

"I have no tongue!" He grunted out in staccato phonemes. Oh. that explains that. Now I felt bad for trying to engage him in conversation. Seems a little bit entitled. Yeah, I know you literally can't speak but I, your humble pizza man, need to perform this small talk. I suddenly had so many questions. Some I would never be allowed to ask, like whether he was born without it or lost it somehow; both stories that would be fascinating, but you're not allowed to interview people about their disabilities unless you're covering the Paralympic Games for a legitimate news organization.

I also had less horrible questions, specifically about the double extra olives. Everyone's got their own taste but people sans tongues, too? And olives but no olive oil? Sprite I get. You can totally taste bubbles, lemon and lime with your nose. But olives are gross and make the entire sandwich feel like an octopus got into it and died. But I digress. And holy shit, he's been talking this whole time, or trying. What the hell is he going on about? He lives here? It's his job to live here? He protects this strip-mall on a dirt island in the flight path of the airport? Protect it from what? Who pays him? What did you study to get that job and why don't you have to wear a shirt to work? Shit man just give me the check so I can go, I'm in way over my head.

He paused long enough for me to agree profusely, a thing I do when I'm done with a conversation that someone is very passionate about, that way they understand that further energy expenditure would be a waste since I'm already on their side and they can stop trying to convince me. The more I want to be out of the conversation the more I'll agree, sometimes going a bit farther than they are just so they get a little bit uncomfortable and end the conversation on their own so rather than being a rude pizza guy I'm a pizza guy with a heart of gold whose only crime is that I believed too much. Marcus smiled, and I gestured back to my car. "Gotta roll, Marcus, two more deliveries in the car." He understood, passed me the check and went back inside. I went right back to the shop. Having lied about the remaining deliveries I just wanted to smoke a cigarette and make some cola wine.

Not all the regulars were weird crazy, some were just crazy crazy. Crazy not in the sense of mental difficulties, but crazy like outrageous! Example: Club 215. It's a strip club near the 215 freeway in Grand Terrace that has parking spots for tractor-trailers and a motel. Once a week we'd get an order from there and all the drivers would fight over who would get to take it if they saw the ticket. If nobody saw it because they weren't snooping, or it was just too busy to look, it was just who was up in the rotation when the order was ready to go. I don't know why everyone was so stoked to make that delivery. The bouncer paid with a twenty and gave you the change which was nothing to turn your head at because a tip is a tip but it's not like you brought the pizza into the champagne room and got to live there for weeks at a time. Three times I didn't even have to get out of my car to make the exchange which felt super drug dealery but was actually remarkably convenient. Dewey said he had to bring wings and breadsticks into the dressing room and was swarmed, but we all know he was full of shit.

There was also the Alano club which had a bunch of coffee cups on the wall with peoples' names on them. They always offered me coffee to go which I always thought was weird because I thought Alano was a pun for the Alamo but in reality, it was short for alcoholics anonymous and I think they knew I was drinking because my entire body was always swollen and sometimes I'd have it on my breath or whatever so good on them.

There was an entire street we wouldn't deliver pizzas to because a couple drivers got robbed so we just cut off the whole street, which is the exact opposite of a regular. My biggest fear was being robbed. I didn't want it to happen at all. I knew I was a total coward, so I didn't want to have to be on the wrong end of a gun, lose all my tips for the night and then have to explain to the police that I had pooped my pants out of fear. I would always promise myself I would write a story about a mysterious stranger, a pizza man with a thousand-yard stare who takes the gun away from his would-be robber and then robs him! Man, that driver would be so cool! What a character! There's nothing else to that story except some lucid violence which always made me feel uncomfortable to think about while outlining the story, so I never followed through with it.

Pre-writing that story, though, was the one thing that kept my mind sharp and my fears at bay while walking through the enormous Peppertree Apartments which were half a block from the robbery street and were rumored by the townies - who would know things like this, to be even sketchier than the robbery street. They were white stucco with green roofs and each of the thirty buildings was four apartments stacked two by two. There was no call box or any other way to get into the complex except to wait out front for someone with a clicker. Once you were in you were trapped until someone opened the gate again; a frightful prospect if you're worried about having to escape, or if you have another delivery to make or want to get back to the shop in a hurry to get as close to the head of the delivery queue as possible because more deliveries mean more money. As far as I knew nothing ever happened to any drivers at Peppertree, but for all intents and purposes it was haunted by the ghosts of potential robbery and that was enough to make it a chore.

The worst regular lived at a confusing address. This delivery trip was always a pain in the ass because streets are remarkably predictable in the way they're set up. If a street has four digits in the addresses it'll be four digits the whole way. Unless of course it's an enormous street then it'll have four digits until 9999 but then it'll roll over instantly to 10000. I don't know of any streets like that specifically but I'm sure they exist somewhere or at least could, as the logic is thorough. This street, however went from the three-hundreds to the fifteen thousands mid-block. I'm sure it has something to do with old timey subdivisions or something stupid, but it was annoying. None of the parallel streets have this sudden jump and nobody else on this rough section ordered pizza consistently enough to expose the rule.

You're driving in your car in your twenties. You've got some thoughts on your mind, a lit cigarette in your hand and the steering wheel in the other. You look at an address and you're a full power of ten away from your intended destination, so you relax and keep on rolling. Two blocks later you're a block too far. Son of a bitch. Turn around! It's fucking Bushnell. You always forget about Bushnell, the regular. You should've known because it's always the same order: medium pizza, large sandwich, extra-large sprite in a cup with no ice plus a cup of ice on the side and a slice of cheesecake.

Soda in cups is always a pain in the ass. No sizes fit in the cup holder in your 97 Toyota Corolla and there's no safe way to transport it outside of a cup holder, so you wedge it among the food as best as you can and hope for the best. That's if you don't forget it completely and have to drive back to the shop to go get it to bring back and make it right. You know if you forget the fountain drink you're ruining someone's night because now they don't have their drink with their dinner, so their mouth is going to be all dry, or they can wait and have cold food. Either way, you're not getting a good tip, not that you deserve one you dang dummy, you forgot the soda!

There are never any cars in this driveway, and never any lights on in the house. No street lights, either. The lawn is dirt and there's some old truck parts around the side probably. There has to be. It's one of those houses. The stoop is cement and unremarkable. The doorbell doesn't work. You have to knock. You have to choose between knocking on the side of the house - stucco, or the fucking dumbass security screen door which somehow both wrecks your knuckles and makes no noise at all. You ball up your fist and bang on the door and now it sounds like you're serving a fucking warrant.

The door opens and the first thing you notice is that it's kind of dark, but the TV is on and throwing enough light into the room to silhouette whoever has opened the door. Then there was the smell: earthy, grassy, salty and poopy; chicken shit. If you've smelled it, you'll remember it forever and can pick it out of a mix of anything. There were no chickens though, ever. The next thing you notice is that silhouette isn't standing at the door, it's sitting. On a bed. There is a bed in the front room and there is a person leaning from it trading you money for food. This person is enormous. This person maybe can't get out of the bed? Maybe this person is too fat to get out of bed, or maybe this person is fat because they can't get out of bed? You're a pizza delivery driver not a doctor but it's not normal. She's nice but you're never able to be as nice as you really are because you are still coming down from getting lost on the way, a bit drunk, and every sense you have is overrun - smell, sight, wonder and balance. I never left that house feeling good. I didn't need to feel good about every delivery, it was just a job, but I also wanted to understand what was happening with that person. I never asked, of course because even I have limits.

The universe is not without a sense of irony, of course, and for all the negative karma I built up rolling through the Alano club drunk, or wondering out loud with the other drivers about the ethics of delivering less than the healthiest food to someone who was bedridden by weight, and making up stories about how Marcus lost his tongue or why he lived in a strip mall, it never really came back in force. There were some rough deliveries, not being able to find the apartment that was "right by the pool," because there were three pools in the goddamn apartment complex, or the guy who tried to get me to join his multi-level-marketing business, or the schools, or the absolute worst: the supermarket runs.

Going to the market as a driver is a pain in the ass. It's a big bright room full of civilians and you're a little sweaty, maybe a bit hungover because they always happened on the morning shift, or maybe you smoked a little pot to take the edge off the hangover and you're in the store and hungry as hell but you're shopping with someone else's money and they're probably not cool with you buying a couple snickers bars or double stuff Oreos or whatever. Plus, even sober and showered, the supermarket is hard. It's a minefield of trick questions and impossible objects. Items of note include Velveeta cheese which is not in the cheese aisle, red onions which are purple but it's easy enough to figure out and also red cabbage which is also purple but there's also sometimes some red stuff nearby that looks like cabbage and that's wrong so if you buy ten pounds of it you'll have to go back and explain to the manager that you bought the wrong thing but ten pounds of it and oh my god does he know I'm high why am I sweating?

There was also nobody to tip you at the supermarket which was a real bummer.

14. "THE BEST SLICE IN LOS ANGELES."

My first job out of college was as a temp. The temp agency I was with catered to mostly entertainment clients. Whenever someone's assistant would go on vacation or catch jury duty or something, they would have a temp cover their desk. To say I had no experience would be exactly true, but for the purpose of this story I will say, "to say I had no experience would be an understatement," because while it is not possible to have less than no experience, an emphatic over exaggeration makes for better reading, and it's totally my style.

I was an awful assistant. I take directions very well, but my judgement is poor in general and was very raw at the time. Therefore, things like when to email your boss, when to interrupt meetings for phone calls, and when to sneak out for a cigarette were not easy and I definitely did them wrong. After my first day on my first assignment they told me what a good job I had done, and that the guy I was replacing had completed his jury service and so I was no longer needed. I knew it was a lie, because I spoke to the assistant throughout the day as he complained about his selection and how long the case was going to take. It was nice that they tried to protect my feelings, but I got the hint instantly and I think that made it hurt a bit more than if I hadn't known the truth.

The next gig was a bit more my speed and required almost no judgment. It was a robotic job - mostly data entry with occasional very long walks to deliver or pick up video tapes. I liked it. I could listen to music and the walks gave me ample opportunity to smoke cigarettes, as well as plausible deniability in case anyone ever was looking for me they would just assume I was out on a delivery or whatever and not be upset that I wasn't at my desk. The job was in a department I had never heard of at one of the best cable networks at the time, which is now inarguably the greatest network of all time. It wasn't a dream gig, though, it was money.

Eventually they offered me the job permanently which included benefits. Since I had a chronic medical condition that made it literally impossible for me to get health insurance without being on a group plan, and with no hopes of making the WGA as I had booked zero writing gigs, I took the job instantly. It was not a sexy job. It was not the job I thought I'd have when I moved to Los Angeles, but it was full time stable work with medical, dental and vision, a pension, a 401k match, in the same industry as my intended career, and with the sole exception of my boss everyone was rad as hell.

The job meant that I didn't have to worry about where my next meal was coming from. It meant that I didn't have to steal my roommate's Lortab (he was recovering from a gnarly motorcycle wreck and had unlimited refills, so I helped myself) to treat the pain in my gut and slow down the diarrhea from the ulcerative colitis. The job meant that I could sign a lease and stop squatting in the frat house in which I was living at the time. The job meant that I could stop trying to survive all the damn time and instead start to enjoy life. I started drinking good beer. Ok I started drinking more shitty beer, but I mean eventually I started drinking good beer, too. Anyway, my life got better instantly, and I had the job to thank.

One day at the job there was a technician there to fix a photocopier because the company that made that particular photocopier refused to let anyone but their own technicians work on the photocopiers that they made. It was near my birthday and my boss and I were talking about which pizza place we were going to get pizzas from for the employee celebration as I had asked for pizza instead of cake. The technician, waiting for something or other decided he wanted to join our conversation.

"You know where the best pizza I've ever had was?" He asked, meaning well, I'm sure.

"Please stop talking," I shot back instantly and probably too loudly as everyone in the office stopped what they were doing and turned their attention to me in the hopes that I would soon provide context for that extremely shitty and totally unprovoked attack on a stranger. I obliged. "I only mean that whatever you think is the best pizza isn't and will only draw rage from me and make me hate you." The context did not improve the situation. He blinked. Jaws slowly lowered around the bullpen. Eyes widened. The man who sat behind me stood up like the manager of a baseball team who knows it's time to pull his pitcher. I could sense my time was limited and I felt the need to further explain, and quickly before someone shut me up. "I only mean that all pizza is good pizza and the love of one is practiced at the expense of all the others!"

Paraphrasing Nietzsche in a panic is not something most production assistants did often, I imagine, so it goes without saying that this story got around the office fairly quickly, or maybe the story was positioned as "can you believe what a giant fucking jerk that Greg kid is?" Either way, it got a lot of heat and increased the traffic to my cubicle. At the time, the network at which I worked was small so the number of people was small, but the percentage of overall employees who had an opinion on pizza was impressive. Everyone, it seemed, had a suggestion for best pizza in Los Angeles.

After a few I started writing them down, if only to spot them as I drove by on my way to some nice restaurant or fancy comedy show or something else. I have the type of synesthesia that makes it, so I orient myself by autobiographical landmarks, so having more things I had heard of definitely gave me more opportunity to feel at home in a city in which I had no experience.

Instead of being in that big expensive gap near Fairfax high school with no parking, it's the neighborhood around Brett's favorite pizza place. If Brett has been here and been cool with it, the neighborhood must be fine and there's probably nothing to be afraid of. I worked with a dude named Brett who really liked Tomato Pie, in case you were wondering what that was about. Instead of thinking my own neighborhood was garbage and a dead zone except for a really awesome Irish dive-bar, I found out that The Coop was a really old and incredibly solid slice shop, cash only, right near an equally random liquor store both of which came highly recommended by one of the guys I smoked cigarettes with who was also my neighbor but whose name I forget. Even the neighborhood where Hoover ends at Wilshire is right near where another coworker (who will remain nameless) got hepatitis, so when I accidentally ended up there late one night, I knew to not stop for pizza (always a struggle for me), and to just keep driving.

A couple months later, and with another Ulcerative Colitis flare raging inside of my guts, my doctor put me on a powerful corticosteroid. This was nothing new, unfortunately, but this cycle was the third cycle in a year and that was uncommon. Steroids are very effective for reducing inflammation which is the root of all the most unpleasant symptoms of ulcerative colitis. These aren't the cool steroids that give you muscles. These are the unfortunately necessary anti-inflammatory medications that are the last line of defense when your body thinks your colon is an infection and attacks it as such.

If you over-use them you could wreck your liver. If you become dependent on them the damage they can cause is less risky than removing your colon. They are not fun. But they are a means to an end of ending the flare and having a life that does not revolve around being very close to a toilet for months at a time. Their downsides include bottomless rage, changing the shape of your face (the fleshy bits under your chin get all enlarged and moon-y), and a hunger that defies description. It is a limitless insatiable hunger that infects every corner of rational thought in every part of your day. Even when you're eating you're starving. You eat so much; your girlfriend will literally cry. Have you ever eaten so much that you made your girlfriend cry?

When you're eating that much, weight gain is unavoidable. I've lost the same thirty to fifty pounds a half a dozen times in my life. I've quit smoking. Nothing has been harder than managing my appetite while on corticosteroids. But you know the saying: when life gives you a chronic condition that can only be treated by intense drugs that make you super hungry, try and find a way to enjoy it. I grabbed that list of best pizza places that I had cobbled from coworkers' suggestions, posted it to Facebook soliciting more opinions, improvements and places to avoid (remember the hepatitis place?), and set off to discover the best piece of pizza in Los Angeles.

This is not a listicle. This isn't ten slices of pizza to try before you die (number four will blow your mind!). This is a fucking memoir. After a year of daily nine out of ten pain, strained relationships and reclusive behavior that were the result of being chained to a toilet, I finally had a silver lining: a call to action. Every weekend I would drive around and hit three to four pizza shops to sample the wares. I would meet people for pizza. I would plan stuff to do with my girlfriend in weird parts of town in order to have an excuse to try a slice.

I explored the city in which I lived with a girl I loved celebrating the best food on earth. I got to know my friends better by trying their favorite of a thing and never got too full for another slice once. On Saturdays, I would even stop on the way home and grab a pie for the night. It was great. Except for the rage and the fact that no matter how much I ate I would never be full. Looking back, this is the year I learned that eating enough and feeling full were distinctly different, and that is the most important lesson anyone who wants to eat nothing but pizza but still lose weight can learn. That and the Vito's white pesto slice will make you slap your mama, it's so fucking good.

15. "STITCHES."

After three weeks of The Great Pizza Experiment I was down almost eight pounds. I was starting to get punchy and cocky. I was seriously in love with cookie shakes and started to add them to lunch instead of just being an evening treat on heavier training days. It got me thinking about dessert once the diet was over and how that would look going forward. I loved ice cream and would probably miss pizza, so I figured pizza ice cream might be something I could get into. Then I said it out loud -- to myself, and as soon as I heard it I thought better of it. Pizza ice cream existed before, I did not invent it. I did, however, have a history of inventing amazing food.

My first true invention was the dojo's daco. I invented it during my fifth year in college when I was living in a house called "the dojo." Actually, it was called "The Eagle's Nest," from the years it housed a fraternity which apparently didn't mind their house sharing a name with Hitler's Bavarian hideaway. My housemates and I very much did mind, so we tried to rebrand it as the dojo, but it never quite took off like we wanted it to. One of the lasting legacies of the name was the snack I invented in the upstairs kitchen (there were two kitchens) (there was also a sauna, a full bar, a spiral staircase and a wraparound patio on the second and third floors) (house was fuckin sweet). The dojo's daco was a hard taco shell with a hotdog in the bottom, two meatballs on top, brown sugar and BBQ sauce. It wasn't pizza, but it was good as fuck.

The next best thing was "the Boytos Pizzarito" which was just a pizza with a tortilla for a crust and then wrapped up. I've never made, nor had one. It came to me in a dream in grad school and after tweeting about it, a colleague from undergrad read it, liked the idea, happened to be a chef and added it to the menu of the restaurant at which he worked while getting his MFA. As his school was on the east coast, I never had the pleasure of trying it, but he said he would run it as a special on the slow days and it did the best between four and four-thirty pm. It was a pizza with a tortilla crust, but the rolling of it removed the pizza from it. It was delicious I'm sure, but it was stromboli, if anything. Not my finest work.

My finest work was the choco-burger. It's a plain cheese burger with chocolate instead of cheese. It came to be when I was in grad school at a fourth of July BBQ. You'll be shocked to know we ran out of cheese. We did have s'mores ingredients laying around, so I got the only melty bit I could from the pile and improvised. We ran out of burgers and chocolate soon after because everyone who took a bite had two full choco-burgers. We had to stumble to the store to get more, and the one thing we didn't re-up on was cheese. It may not have been pizza, but it'll make somebody famous someday.

They're not all hits though: my food inventions. Emboldened by the runaway success of the chocolate burger and a fond memory of the dojo's daco from the year before, I invented the biggest flop of my food inventing career the very week after creating the choco-burger. The choco-dog. A hotdog with melted chocolate as the sauce. Woof. I'm sorry for ever mentioning it. It's probably as bad as pizza ice cream would be though, which is how I started down this whole road to begin with.

For the great pizza experiment, I was limited to milkshakes and dessert pizza which were enough. Dessert pizza is fantastic. My favorite recipe used butter as the sauce and a flour, cinnamon and sugar mix for the cheese. It was gritty in the best way. As soon as you felt the mix between your teeth the butter and heat and your saliva melted it all together and the grit would disappear into sweet and savory magic. Since The Great Pizza Experiment has ended I have discovered a s'mores pizza which is superior to this. The sauce is chocolate and the cheese is marshmallows. It's a thing of true beauty and the only bad thing about it is that I didn't invent it.

This being the fourth week, my new diet had become a habit. It was still amazing, but it wasn't work anymore. It wasn't new anymore. I burned no calories trying to figure out what to eat for lunch, and only had to consider where I would order pizza from. In a worst-case scenario where I couldn't decide, there was even a decent spot at work. I usually liked to go with leftovers on days where I trained immediately before breaking my fast, but on days where I trained in the morning or rest days or days where I knew I'd be pulling a double in the evening, I could go explore. Since I'm a boring man, exploring means going to a place kind of far away over and over again.

That place was 800 degrees pizza. They had a deal Monday through Friday called the pizza of the day where they posted a pizza on Instagram and if you wanted it in that exact configuration, it'd be only five bucks. If it sucked I would skip it, but I like most pizza, so I was there more often than I wasn't. Since I was splitting my time between two offices at the time, luck provided an 800 degrees pizza near enough to each to make it my number one spot. I saved the number in my phone as "bae," and since I hate talking on the phone so much, there were some weeks when the only calls in my history were missed incoming calls and outgoing calls to bae.

I felt so good on the diet. Workouts were exhausting but I would recover easily and be able to go again almost instantly. I was sleeping through the night and waking up before my alarm clock with energy and excitement. Things were clicking and rolling and floating and sailing. It was one of those rare points of my life where I achieved total clarity of purpose. It was like a macro flow state. I've never even heard about a thing like that, but I was living it. It was glorious.

Tuesday of week four I ran before lunch, crushed a pizza of the day and worked a little later than normal. I got home just as it was getting dark and set up my work out. It was a simple workout with kettlebell swings, kettlebell snatches and box jumps. I set it up like a circuit rotating through each move and doing it as many times as I could in forty seconds then resting for twenty before moving onto the next move. It would go on like that for thirty minutes. It would go on like that, except on the third round of box jumps I shorted one, kicked the box and slammed my shin down on the corner of the box. Gravity dragged me down a couple inches before I was able to catch myself with my hands and push off.

It hurt but I didn't even look at it. I set my feet took a breath and jumped again. When I landed on top of the box I saw a lot of blood on my white shoe and a fair amount of blood, skin and hair on the corner of the box. The world flashed white and I realized this could be a real hurt. I looked at my shin. I have a tattoo on the side of my calf of a little devil -- my dad has the same one and one year my brother and I each got a copy of one of our dad's tattoos. I got the devil and he got the skunk from Bambi. Anyway, my devil is holding a pitchfork and right at the end of the pitchfork was an inch-long gash revealing bone and pouring blood into my sock.

The world flashed white again. I'd never seen my shin before. I took a breath and sat down. I was bleeding profusely. It looked bad. My first thought: stop the bleeding so I can finish the workout. I ran inside and grabbed a paper towel and a handkerchief and made a little MacGyver bandage. It soaked through before I was finished tying it. I got a couple more paper towels and applied pressure, but they soaked through soon as well. This was bad. I took a picture and texted it to my friend, Toby who I try to maintain a relationship with by sending dumb or gross texts, and his college roommate Amit, who is a doctor.

Toby didn't react in any major way, just asked a bunch of context questions. Amit told me it was not my shin I was seeing, but fascia, a bit of tissue between your muscle and skin to keep things tight. That was good. He said I should get stitches though, as shin wounds tend to be notoriously bad at healing. I've never had stitches before, so I didn't know what to expect. had been admitted to the hospital twice, once while pissing blood from rhabdo and another time while vomiting bile and hallucinating from ulcerative colitis induced dehydration and malnutrition, but I had never had stitches and I had never gone in alone.

I hatched a plan to wait for my wife to get home and have her take me to urgent care. By the time she got there, urgent care was closed so we had to go to the emergency room. The problem with having an urgent care level injury in an emergency room is that everyone else goes before you. We got there at 9:15 but didn't get in to see the doctor until close to one in the morning. Every nurse commented on how well the divot fit my tattoo, though, so I knew I was somehow a little lucky. Eight stitches later and they sent me home.

The next day it hurt to walk. Exercising was out of the question. Boredom set in rapidly. When I get bored I get depressed, so I was bracing myself for that, but it never came. It turns out when you eat nothing but pizza you can't get depressed. Consuming nothing but the magical ratio of bread to sauce to cheese alters your dopamine receptors to such an extent that you are depression proof. Instead of feeling bored then sad, I felt bored then inspired. I spent my entire lunch break either napping or making pizza films - two of the noblest art forms.

Calling what I made "films" would be being very generous. I made short, pointless, self-indulgent videos of pizza. I would shoot a slow-motion video of me taking a wicked bite, a reverse video of me taking a bite, or a stop motion video of me taking a bite. I didn't find every way to shoot myself taking a bite, but I tried my best and I didn't want to make just video anyway because I was filing everything away on the hashtag #pizzatos (pizza + Boytos) so I could review my legacy after the experiment if I was ever bored or sad or whatever. I figured future me would want some mixed media. I was right. Reviewing the hashtag while writing this book I'm glad I didn't just make a ton of stupid videos and took some stupid pictures as well.

Another weird thing about having eight stitches in your shin is that you know what touches the inside of your pants with every step? Your shin. So, once the numbing agent wears off the twine they use to close your skin brushes up against grabby thick cloth about five thousand times a day. It's absolutely as strange and unnerving as you would imagine. When the pain wore off there was still a ton of swelling which had its own fresh collection of discomfort.

I wore shorts to work. I was working off-site on this day and didn't think it'd be a big deal because my boss never stopped by. It ended up being fine, professionally. I didn't get in trouble, at least. It felt so gross to be doing work things in work spaces with other people who were working while I was wearing shorts. Seeing your coworkers' legs is weird. They're always the wrong color and with an alarming amount of hair or not nearly enough. That day I was that guy. I had a good excuse, but I still didn't like everyone being able to see my legs. As a compromise, I started wearing a bandage on the stitches to keep them from rubbing the inside of the pant leg.

With all the rest of the free time I saved not being able to work out, I had time to dream a little bit. I started thinking of ways to keep this going for as long as possible. I had already worked in a pizza shop and didn't hate it, but there was a ceiling there under which I wasn't comfortable. Owning a pizza shop was also an option but I lacked the capitol, the expertise, and the opportunity. Then I wrote down "president of pizza," in my notebook and about a thousand hearts like I was a twelve-year-old girl. None of those are real jobs though. Not really, anyway, the only one I could realistically do I'd already done, and I know what it paid so I didn't need to do it again. Not that I'm above washing dishes, but it's not very presidential, and I had a job already, so it was not really an issue. I don't need to explain myself to you.

In between dreams and epiphanies pizza memories began flooding back. Because I'm Italian, though, the first memory that came flooding back was a grudge. It was about this thing called "The Pizzafest." Danny DeVito was supposed to be there or something, which made it very obviously legit and awesome. Part all you can eat pizza cafe, part pizza ted talk, trade show, samples and instant membership in the fraternal order of pizza. I spent two hours' pretax salary on a ticket! I looked forward to it for over a month. I cancelled plans for it. I skipped dinner the night before and breakfast on the day of.

I arrived and there was a line. Lines are the worst invention I've ever heard of, but they're inevitable at cool shit like the Pizzafest. There were two lines, actually, one general admission line and one VIP line. The general

THE GREAT PIZZA EXPERIMENT

admission line was long, and the VIP line was short, but something about how fast the general admission line moved made me think the festival was less mismanaged than it was. I got through the queue, was given a commemorative wine glass and sent inside immediately. Which was cool. I had made it. I was inside.

Inside was great! Inside was where all the pizzas were! There was so much pizza that the entire room smelled like pizza, which is my favorite smell. There were lines everywhere though. So many lines from booth to booth and table to table and even one that stretched all the way out the door. When does a line ever go from inside to outside?! This place must be amazing! All the pizza was so good that the whole dang place was just lines. I wanted to grab a slice but had to select the line that would be the best! Spoiler alert: all of the lines led to pizza and they moved slow. As. fuck. Danny DeVito never showed up. There were no pizza TED talks. There isn't a pizza fraternity at all and if there was one, they wouldn't be caught dead at this debacle.

The Pizzafest was six hours long but after I spent two hours in pizza lines, the second of which ended with a half of a piece of Digiorno supreme pizza on a napkin. The wine glass lay empty in the reusable shopping bag they gave us at some point. I walked out, paid for parking, grabbed a couple of large pizzas from a local spot and cry ate until I was full and empty at the same time.

The goddamn scam of scams. It was the Fyre festival of pizza, if people at the Fyre festival liked a good thing like pizza and not a shitty thing like whatever the fuck was supposed to happen at the Fyre festival. I was livid for weeks and I refuse to drink out of the shitty wine glass that I keep in my cabinet as a reminder not to be a shitty dickhead like the planners of the Pizzafest. At the time of writing it was eight years ago and I've had to take three breaks to breathe deep and recover my center, so the cut was and is deep and I never want to forget the pain.

I had lost it. Remembering the Pizzafest made me see red. Thanks to my swollen, sutured shin, I couldn't even work out the rage in a productive manner, so I had to sit back and tough it out. I went a little bit crazy. I thought I was pizza. I could feel myself melting and bubbling and sweating, browning and delicious. I tagged myself in a bunch of strangers' pizza pictures on social media. People do not react well to strange dudes declaring that they are pizza.

The fourth week of The Great Pizza Experiment left me broken and battered. I couldn't move, and I couldn't get anything moving. I never lost enthusiasm for The Great Pizza Experiment, but the fact remained that I had become quite accustomed to a high calorie diet based around vigorous exercise and the injury prevented that transaction from benefiting me. That said, I did not gain a single ounce, but instead ended the week the exact same weight as when the week started. Call it dumb luck or whatever you like but having a same weight week to week even during non-experimental dieting is incredible. The other incredible thing about having the stitches in my shin was that I could control the weather. Which was nice.

16. "RHABDO."

I ran my first half marathon with my wife in the year 2011. Before training for that race, I had never run more than four miles at a time. The way to train for a half marathon is to progressively increase your mileage until you can run about ten miles, then you take a couple weeks to taper your mileage down before your race and then on race day you're trained and rested and can finish. Using this method, I set new personal records for total distance run in a single run almost every week for eight weeks in a row.

It felt good to run farther than I ever had. It is beyond explanation. Sometimes I would cry as I eclipsed the previous record and began the record-setting mile. It also felt good to work out four times a week and know what every workout had to accomplish. Training programs for running are very satisfying in a box-checking way, the same way a to-do list makes you feel more productive. On day one you know what you had to accomplish every day of every week for the next twelve weeks in a row and if you took it bit by bit and stayed on task you would make tremendous progress. The accomplishing thing was probably more satisfying for me than progressively increasing mileage, but they were both incredible feelings for me, a former fat kid who was unable to run a continuous mile in P.E. class in high school. The focus point of the training week was the weekend long run. This run was the one that inspired the weekly celebration, marked the progress you had made and the improvement week to week you were making as a distance runner. Each week this long run was celebrated with pizza, for me. It was my cheat meal. The meal that didn't count as far as calories, even though a five-mile run is hardly enough to earn a true pizza gorge fest.

During the second half of my training cycle, my best friend told me he was running the San Francisco Marathon which was the perfect number of weeks after my half marathon to continue my training trajectory and toe the line alongside him in whatever San Francisco's nickname is -- probably something dumb like The Golden Gate City. He just shrugged and said it fit into the schedule. He was so nonchalant about it that I believed him. This was before I realized how much of a remarkable salesperson he was, so I had no reason to not believe him. He was not wrong, because I did continue my training trajectory and I did make it to the start line healthy and in shape. He did not, however, as he couldn't make the time commitment to training because of his success as an in-demand salesperson. I would not have run the race without his suggestion, though, so in a way most of my running disease is his fault. Did you read that Thomas Roy Littlejohn? This is on you.

The race was fine, but my official finish time and my goal time were so far apart that I could not be happy with just finishing. Don't get me wrong, I openly wept at several points during the race and was overcome with emotions at the finish when I saw my girlfriend (now wife) among the crowd of strangers cheering for me despite my slow-ish time. I was happy with the finish, but I was not content. I had unfinished business.

After the race, I went out for pizza. Surprised? We went to little Italy in San Francisco and ate Roman style pizza which was a genuine treat. It was my first time having Roman style pizza, it's square and thin and pizza so it's perfect. The best part of the meal was the proprietor of the pizza shop. She was graceful, welcoming and charming in a way I'd only seen within my close-knit family and San Biagio, something that could only happen in a pizza shop. Every other restaurant is too cold, and a pizza shop is warm in a way that only home can be.

Despite the belly full of pizza, I was hungry. Not for more food though if there was more pizza I could've eaten, but for a better result. I had started the race at two-hundred and seventeen pounds which was heavy. read a statistic that every pound lost results in a two second improvement per mile at the same effort so to accomplish my goal of a sub-four-hour marathon, I would need to lose sixty pounds. That was too much weight to lose. I would just have to train harder and smarter!

I read Born to Run and decided that barefoot running was the way to go. Not barefoot without shoes, because I don't think that is wise, nor did I want to be that guy. I bought new shoes -- barefoot shoes that protect the feet from the cruel world but allow them to function as if they were unshod, not the goofy toe-shoes that your weird neighbor wears to the apple store, either. These looked like normal shoes. I spent six months training my stride. I trained hard, set a new half-marathon PR and was primed for another marathon with excellent fitness and ten fewer pounds when I picked up a stress fracture in my foot and ended the season.

I had joked for weeks about having something rattling around in my foot, and then on my last long run before the marathon the soreness was overwhelming, and I finished but couldn't walk without a limp. I was at the beach, so I stood in the water for twenty minutes hoping the ocean temperature in March would be low enough to knock down the inflammation and keep me running, but it was not to be. I was in a walking boot by lunch the next day and it'd be six weeks before I could start running again.

In that six weeks of forced rest I conducted a thorough investigation of what went wrong in my foot. It seemed that I had increased distance too fast for barefoot running. It was my own fault. Another magic bullet fitness fad that failed me personally and the conventional wisdom was that it was user error. I was so used to it at this point that it didn't even sting. Running barefoot was supposed to make me a stronger, faster, more efficient runner and instead it broke my foot and made me unable to run at all. It seems as if my weight -- lower than before but still high, was an issue. So was the surface I chose to run on.

Running on roads can be rough on your joints. Running on trails is not as rough on them. Running trails that most people hike, though, is difficult and scary to begin. While I was healing I started to read up on trail running. There was a ton of information out there and I went down a rabbit hole of blogs and social media. There was a whole bunch of people running on dirt through the mountains around the world, and they were not stopping at the end of a marathon. They would run ultramarathons of fifty kilometers, fifty miles, one hundred kilometers, one hundred miles and more!

I had never considered anything as insane as running over a hundred miles for fun. I never thought running one mile was fun but the sense of accomplishment after was addicting. People talk about runner's high but I'm not sure those people have ever done real drugs. I never got high once from running and that is the truth. I loved the way that pizza tasted after I got home, though, and the way the beer tasted in the shower the afternoon after running twenty miles, too. The rest of the day after a long morning run you're this dream sequence of heavy feet and sore quads. You just float around knowing that the hardest part of your day is over. You can do anything, and nobody can call you lazy because you already ran twenty dang miles! And if that was true for marathons, it must be ultra-true for ultramarathons!

I bought an ultrarunning book and as soon as I could run again I was back at it. The training cycle was six months long, so I picked a nearby race seven months in the future and devised a training plan. I trained five days a week all winter, rain or shine, hangover or not. I skipped social functions, eschewed vacations, ignored family and ran, ran, ran. I was right. The pizza tasted better after longer runs at the end of high mileage weeks. I ate so much pizza after my runs that I did not lose a single pound despite spending ten to twelve hours per week running.

When race day arrived, I had my usual pre-run breakfast: matzo brei. I was a little concerned that after a very mild Southern California winter where the high temperature never got above the low seventies, the high for race day was in the upper eighties, but I reasoned aloud, "just drink more water." I was nervous about the race in the starting chute, but not anything about racing. Every start line is full of the same anxiety for me, so much so that I have a mantra. "I just hope I don't shit my pants."

THE GREAT PIZZA EXPERIMENT

The gun went off and hundreds of strangers set off to run fifty kilometers through the foothills of Simi Valley, CA. I chose a fifty kilometer for my first ultra because the prevailing wisdom was that your increases should come in increments and every new race distance was a completely different beast, full of lessons that you would need to get through the next one. I've heard the fifty-kilometer distance referred to as "the diet ultra," but I've never heard anyone who's run a single ultra disparage the distance the way my shitty coworkers do.

The race was going fine for the first ten miles. I was moving slower than I had planned because of the heat, but I was also drinking extra water, so it evened out. I also stepped up my salt cap ingestion from one every forty minutes to one every thirty minutes. I run with a race vest, which is essentially a tiny backpack full of water with extra straps to keep the water bladder from bouncing around as you run. There's a long straw that connects to this water to your mouth and there's pockets everywhere to carry extra calories, cell phones, emergency blankets and anything else you want to carry.

The vest carries two liters of water and with my heat mitigation strategy, I had drunk it all over the first ten miles. When I got to an aid station -- a checkpoint on the race course staffed with dozens of the friendliest, most accommodating, helpfullest runners who have taken the day from running or racing to help you accomplish your goals, a man offered to fill my pack. I let him do it as I grazed the checkpoint's legendary food table full of gummy bears, Oreos, pretzels, peanut butter sandwiches, and other caloric density foods. He gave me my pack back and I took off. It was five miles to the next aid station, up and over a peak that rose a further thousand feet toward the hot sun. As I cruised into the next aid station I heard the tell-tale bubble noise that indicated my backpack was out of water, so I had them refill it before turning back. Total water consumed: 4 ters. Total distance so far: 15 miles.

The race was half over, and I was feeling good. It was undoubtedly hot, but I was crushing water and moving slowly but evenly. The finish line was back through the aid station on the other side of the hill from where I just came, so I set about climbing back over it. About half way up I heard the bubbles again. Out of water. I remember being amazed and doing the math. I had consumed six liters of water in seventeen or eighteen miles, that's a lot of water. By the time I got back to the first aid station I was nauseous. Of course, I was nauseous, I had hyponatremia from drinking way too much water.

I was too nauseous to eat or drink, but I figured since I was hyponatremic I could just hike it off. I pushed on and hiked the last twelve miles to the finish, through the heat so extreme that the race organizers had hired a search and rescue team to roam the course and check on racers. My nausea never improved. I knew I was in trouble when I finished and the volunteer at the finish line offered me pizza and I said, "no thanks." I went and told a medic about my plight, but they were packing up and said I'd be fine.

It was hard driving myself home. The nausea made my head a little dizzy and I felt dissociated, like my eyes were disconnected from my brain and the world was on tape delay. When I got home I forced down a quart of electrolyte drink and hopped in the shower. Normally after hot runs I would grab a shower beer, but I was not feeling well at all, so I skipped it. I had the sudden urge to pee and I was too tired to hold it, so I let it go. It smelled like coffee. Sometimes my pee smells like coffee, but only if it's the first pee after I've drank coffee.

I hadn't had coffee since the cup I drank on the way to the race that morning at four am. I was out on the course for eight hours forty-five minutes and six seconds, drank six liters of water and one quart of electrolyte drink and had not peed once. For someone self-diagnosed with hyponatremia, not peeing at all was not right. Usually you keep peeing until your system evens itself out. This must mean I was dehydrated. I went to check my race vest to re-do the math on how much water I'd ingested and when I opened up the back I noticed the bladder - the place that holds the water, had been twisted.

There was no way to keep the bladder from collapsing on itself in the pack due to a design flaw and with all the jostling that comes with trail running and having multiple people help you fill it up, it got twisted. This means I only had three liters of water, which over a nine-hour adventure in random ninety-degree heat in the middle of a cool winter, is not enough. I had been so dehydrated that I was cognitively compromised blamed my nausea on too much water and stopped drinking which made things so much worse.

Knowing this I started forcing down electrolyte drink despite my nausea. What should've been an evening of beer and pizza and celebration was suddenly a flush fluids on the couch and feel sorry for myself night. The only saving grace was the 2-on-1 date on that night's episode of the bachelor. It is one of the most hyped episodes of every season because it's usually the villain and their main adversary and they face off right in front of the person whose love they're competing to win. The rule of the 2-on-1 date is that one of the competitors will be going home, so there's a guaranteed breakup and the two women - Ashley I and Kelsey, were super volatile and promised a major fireworks show.

Nothing was going to keep me from missing this episode, especially not an upset stomach! When I got up to go pee again, I was relieved. Peeing twice in an hour was proof I was recovering from the dehydration from earlier in the day. I was excited to pee and grab a beer, so I didn't have to waste any more time drinking non-alcoholic stuff; I was a goddamn ultramarathoner now, I had to celebrate my new life! When the pee came out of my penis looking like Coca-Cola, the fear was cloaked in disappointment.

Rhabdomyolysis is blood toxicity caused by muscle breakdown. Muscle breakdown is inevitable in ultramarathons. The idea is to limit it as much as you can with fitness, nutrition and hydration. During cold weather, your body carries less blood volume, making your winter blood a bit thicker than normal. When you're dehydrated that blood volume is further decreased, giving some of its volume to sweat to keep you cool. When you run downhill your legs do about a hundred and eighty eccentric muscle contractions per minute. Eccentric muscle contractions are when the muscles lengthen under a load and are potentially very damaging to the muscle fiber. When you combine all this, you have a sludge made of myoglobin going through the kidneys or trying. This is toxic on its own and can also cause kidney failure. The symptoms of rhabdo include coca cola colored urine and elevated creatinine levels in your blood.

After I peed the blood I was scared, disappointed, and ashamed. Sad because I knew I was in danger, disappointed because I knew people are shitty and would take any opportunity to whisper about me, how I was too underprepared, overweight, or naive to attempt an ultramarathon, and ashamed because maybe they were right. I said to my wife "Hey, after this we have to go to the ER. I have rhabdo." and ninety minutes later, after BOTH Ashley and Kelsey got sent home - yes a rare double breakup on the 2-on-1 date that was so worth it, we were on our way to the same ER would end up in seven months later during The Great Pizza Experiment.

I gave them a urine sample and the nurse took one look and said "yup, that's rhabdo!" They gave me a bed and an IV and a lot of medicine. Medicine for the nausea, medicine to replace the low potassium and magnesium that was altering my heartbeat and some fluids to get some volume in my veins. I was in acute kidney failure due to rhabdomyolysis but there was no medicine for that, only fluids and rest. They admitted me to the hospital and sent my wife home for the night. I had a hard time sleeping as my cardiovascular fitness gave me a resting heart rate well below the alarm setting on the EKG I was attached to, so whenever I got close to zonking out it would blast off and wake me up. When I asked the nurses to change it, that I was an athlete and the low resting heart rate was because was in excellent physical shape, they'd take a quick look at my gut, change nothing and leave the room.

My parents came the next day and the nurse gave them a good scare. They joined the staff on the floor in being very concerned about my decision-making abilities. Why would anyone run longer than a marathon? It's the same dumb thought process that leads strangers to warn you how running ruins your knees. It's not true. It's just something weak people say when they sense you getting away. It's like the townie mentality where they talk shit about their friends in med-school from their parents' basement. It bothers me from an epistemological perspective. Running is good for you. Full stop. Kidney failure is bad for you, though, so I didn't fight.

The groupthink during my four days in the hospital was how lucky I was to be alive and not on dialysis for the rest of my life. They were right. I was very lucky. Then they all started asking me if I learned my lesson. I had to admit that I did, indeed, learn my lesson. I vowed on that day, from that hospital bed in that Kaiser Permanente that I would never run another ultramarathon again, without eating an all pizza diet in the twenty-four hours before the race.

I have kept that vow and it has served me incredibly well. I've run three more fifty-kilometer races with respectable times and a fifty-mile race which I was just glad to finish. I've gotten so serious about this pre-race ritual that it has permeated into most of the athletic endeavors with which I participate. I set a thirty-minute marathon PR on Round Table in Big Sur. I shaved ten more off on Costco frozen pizza in Santa Clarita. I finally broke four hours with Pizza Hut on the famous Los Angeles Stadium to the Sea course. I ate Little Caesars, Lamonica's and Pizza My Heart for a Spartan trifecta, and overcame a panic attack in the first leg of my first triathlon to finish in the top half of the field with Dough Girl pumping through my veins. I've squatted three hundred pounds with a belly full of pizza, deadlifted four hundred, bench pressed a shockingly small amount when compared to the other two, but I'm working on it, give me a break.

17. "DRIVEBY."

When I was a kid I had an allowance. I don't remember how much it was, but it was pretty small. Somehow during the summer, though for whatever reason, I'd have more money. I'd always have walk around money, either from my birthday, or some bullshit scam my best friend and I would pull on the neighbors by collecting stuff in an old box-lid and selling it door to door, or a couple summers when my sister started paying me cash for good grades. And please believe you know where all of that money went: baseball cards and pogs.

Baseball cards were essentially collectible photos and statistics printed on glossy cardboard and sold in packs of about fifteen and one slice of terrible, always stale, chalky bubblegum. The valuable and most desirable cards were the ones featuring the best most popular players or the cards that had errors or some crazy feature that you'd have to see to believe. One guy wrote, "fuck face," or something on the butt of his bat and it got printed so there's a ton of cards from the first half of that year – until the baseball card suits reprinted them with the cuss words cropped out.

Pogs were circular cardboard things that started out as milk caps from Hawaii or something. There was a game -- that we weren't allowed to play because it was technically gambling, that involved the pogs and slammers and you could flip them over and somehow win. Like I said, wasn't allowed to play because it was gambling so I never bothered to learn the rules. I just collected the pogs and the slammers because, honestly, think they were next to the baseball cards and that's how marketing works on young kids with money.

My best friend and I would ride our bikes a mile or two down the hill to the nice pizza place. I don't want to name names, but it was a chain that was medieval themed in its title and décor, and it was, and remains the most expensive chain of pizza of which I am aware. That didn't matter, though, because they had a lunch special: a personal pizza and a soda with unlimited refills for three bucks. They also had a big tv that had baseball games all day, comfortably padded bench seats, and best of all video games.

They had fighting games. They had that game with the trucks where you raced around a dirt track and could buy supplies for your truck between turns. They had that game with the cowboys where each one was a different color and they all had different weapons. They had the games with the guns where you killed aliens. They had everything they needed to get our money and they were efficient. I am not complaining. Games are entertainment and I was entertained. After our lunch and soda bacchanal we would walk next door to the trading card and pog store to let the food settle. Unless we were in the market for a specific card or pog and budgeted our gameplay to allow for an extra purchase, or were particularly flush with cash post birthday, we would just browse and make sure there was nothing we needed to save up for.

One day the store was closed with everything inside. Apparently, the owners' kid drove the getaway car in a drive-by shooting that resulted in the death of a kid in the next town over and either to pay for his legal fees or just because our town was so tiny and up in everyone else's shit they were shamed out of their business or there was a vicious letter printed in the town paper, or something similarly small towny, it closed suddenly. It was replaced by a karate studio, which was not a good place to hang out with a gut full of pizza. We stopped riding our bikes down there after that. We still had money though, so we would just play games at one of our houses and get pizza delivered. That way we could swim, too.

By the time high school rolled around, I lived way on the other side of town. There was a girl that worked at this same pizza place and she had a crush on one of my friends. It was such a hard crush that he somehow parlayed it into incredibly cheap pizza. I'm talking five bucks for an extra-large pizza. That summer we went there every night for two weeks straight and ate like kings. The place started to feel like home.

I first realized that I was a coward there. We were sitting outside waiting for the rest of our friends to show up when a kid from a couple towns over got out of his car and headed to the ice cream shop next door. He had to walk past us to get there, and we were kind of milling about on either side of the path, so he had to walk in between us. This kid was a monster. Six-foot-ten-inches tall and at least three hundred pounds. He was a football player, heavily recruited and known to most of the people our age in the area. He was a bit of a celebrity.

We didn't see him at first, but when we did we couldn't help but stare. He had two friends with him and he was wearing a cowboy hat and cotton underwear briefs. If there's one thing I know now, it's that dudes dressed like that with fully clothed friends in tow, two towns over from where they live, are almost certainly hoping to be stared at so they can start a fight. I saw him, and my eyes got huge and I looked away instantly. Unfortunately, my friend did not have the same instinct and looked right at this guy's junk undoubtedly flopping around in the nut huggers he was tucked into.

The guy boomed some homophobic epithet at my friend, and even though it was still the early twenty-aughts and calling someone gay or a fag was generally accepted, I had a gay family member and had a bit of an education on why using hate speech that included quality judgments about someone's lifestyle was unacceptable. But I said nothing because: coward. He got in my friend's face, which was definitely a sight because at six-foot-four and two hundred twenty pounds, my friend wasn't small, but this guy made him look microscopic. The huge dude was yelling at my friend and his friends were behind him egging him on, and I was trying to disappear like the kids in Jurassic Park. If I don't move, this T-rex of a man wouldn't be able to see me.

In hindsight, getting my friend's back would have escalated things to a fight we certainly would have lost, but at the moment I was not thinking "do not escalate," I was thinking, "don't move. this is very bad but maybe if you freeze they'll only beat up your friends." I can't say what would've happened had there been a fight, but I probably would have weaseled out somehow as I have several times since but due to my lack of action. Thanks to my friend explaining that "of course we're looking at you, you're outside in underwear," and being pretty chill about not laughing in this giant's face, there was no fight. My yellow belly was not revealed to my friends, or they never mentioned it out of shame, or it was just common knowledge that I was a big ole wuss. They were hateful, small town losers looking for trouble and any excuse to use their one advantage to make other people feel bad and potentially do them harm because. Now he's a bouncer at a strip club and I eat pizza for a living. Cowards inherit the earth.

I've been back since I moved away, and the place still has a lot of memories for me. Though they've since pulled down all the medieval chandeliers and replaced the armor, shields and swords with framed prints of armor, shields and swords; though the wood paneled walls have been painted over; the soda is no longer free refills and the games have changed, it still feels more familiar – I hesitate to use the phrase "like home," here – than any other place that I have access to. It seems silly to feel nostalgia for a pizza place and I agree, but sometimes feelings are silly. Any place can hold fond memories for a person and this place is definitely one of those places for me.

18. "CHEAT DAY."

After four weeks of The Great Pizza Experiment I was down a total of eight pounds, but the fourth week yielded no additional losses due to a vicious and unlucky plyo box incident that resulted in a shin full of stitches. This led to boredom and too much free time as I healed. But I was healing. Faster than normal, perhaps, because of my diet?

I went to the wound care facility, so they could inspect my stitches and take them out if possible. The nurse said it was too soon to remove them but remarked at how perfectly aligned the wound was in relation to the tattoo of a devil I have on my shin and complimented the cleanliness of my wound. She didn't ask how I kept it so clean or inquire about my diet, but I told her anyway, "thank you. It's clean because I'm actually eating nothing but pizza." she did that fake smile thing where she basically just showed her teeth and hoped I stopped talking.

"Come back next week and we'll take all seven stitches out." Another sandwicher I'd bet, or maybe she just didn't understand that I was eating only pizza. Also, did she say seven stitches?

"Uh. did you say seven stitches?"

"yes."

"There's eight."

"What?"

"There's eight stitches in my shin."

She looked again. Shook her head. "I'm only seeing seven." she looked at my chart, looked at the shin again. "Maybe the devil ate it." she laughed. "Chart says seven, too." Dang. I only had seven stitches, not eight. Did that make the injury less badass? I hope not because it hurt like hell and was a major inconvenience. I needed pizza.

I went to Westwood village - a college town style neighborhood in Los Angeles that serves UCLA, for some post wound inspection pizza. It's a mini downtown area and along with that comes parking problems. Parking complications would be a better way to say it, as it's never a problem but it's always complicated. You just pull into the village and take the first spot you see and walk from there. Some people like to try and find a close spot, but I outgrew that hope soon after moving there.

There's never any shortage of sidewalk activity, as it goes with most college towns, and I'm usually pretty good about avoiding it. This day I had to choose between a ranting bum and a tent of unassuming looking hippies, so I chose the hippies. They weren't just hippies, they were LaRouche Democrats. As soon as I saw the sign I knew I chose wrong. I mean, they're harmless, they're just annoying. They speak English but it's another language. I understand every word but not what they're saying at all.

I don't even remember what they say or how they say it I just remember confusion. Pure confusion. They raise their voices out of passion and they genuinely believe what they're saying. Starvation, a train, LaRouche but he's dead, I think so there's someone else? I genuinely can't keep up. I can't keep it together. I must escape but they're so nice and they're all in on this movement. I can't give money I don't have. I won't give support to something I can't pretend to understand. I thanked them and wished them luck and went on my way.

I rounded the last corner before the pizza shop and just about crashed into a DARE booth. DARE is an anti-drug program aimed at young people. I never liked it growing up. It always felt like they were lying to us. As a kid, once I figured someone was lying, I lost trust in them completely. A cop taught the class and cops only understand the bad parts of drugs, which are many, but that's the only perspective they have. I knew drugs were bad but I also figured they were sweet because so many people did them, so the fact that the cop wouldn't acknowledge that made me distrust him.

The DARE people, though, were not cops. They were just another group of people out for my attention, support, and money. For whatever reason, I am unable to walk past people who are trying to get my attention without acknowledging them and at least giving a partial explanation. Usually it's "I'm sorry I don't have any cash," to a bum or "I can't vote, I'm a felon," to a signature collector, but with the DARE people I just said, "but I like drugs."

I should've just walked past and not said anything, but instead I was honest. I do like drugs. They work. Sometimes they work too well and break everything else, so I get it, but sometimes, too they're just rad. "We're not against pot, anymore." I stopped. I should've kept walking, but I stopped. Was I now going to pitch this kid on pills or mushrooms or amphetamines? That'd be a weird conversation, sure, but not as weird as "really? Well pot's not a drug, anyway," a weird pause and then, "but. Cool. I was just on my way to eat pizza." and then I walked into the pizza shop.

On the way back to my car I crossed the street early to avoid the LaRouche kids because surely the bum would have moved on by now. I have nothing against bums, in fact I avoid them out of shame. We failed them and I am powerless to help. Their suffering makes me feel feckless and out of pure vanity I choose not to interact. I vote for anything to help them and think something ought to be done, but that's a societal thing, not a person to person thing. In any case, the bum was still there on my way back to the car, but he was surrounded by college kids in matching t-shirts. They were holding hands and bowing their heads, praying? "Leave 'em alone!" I said as I walked past and one of the kids shouted back.

"He's not bothering us. We're praying!"

"I wasn't talking to him," and by the time I got that out they were behind me. All the money churches take in order to provide for those less fortunate and there's still people sleeping on the street. The pope's got a entire city leafed in gold stolen over the years from all around the world and here's people who can't afford long term medical care and are dumped on kid row to fend for themselves. It's shameful and disgusting. Pray all you want but don't lie about wanting to help people. Lack of exercise, it turned out, made me more agro than usual. I was anxious and more willing to shout at praying strangers with all the energy a belly full of pizza provided. I needed this shin thing to wrap up quick!

The next day I drove across town for lunch -- pizza, with a friend. I rarely eat lunch with other people, but The Great Pizza Experiment made people want to eat with me, to see if it were real, maybe? I rarely ate lunch with anybody because nobody ever invites me to lunch. Everyone agrees when I invite them to lunch, but my phone never rings. This experiment was making me a little celebrity and I was soaking it up, even if it meant driving from century city to Burbank and back, which doesn't look far on a map, but it is. For lunch it is an eternity, it just goes to show how eager I am to eat with other people.

That Saturday was my future brother in law's bachelor party down in San Diego. It was a scheduled cheat day, and I like him and his friends, so I was looking forward to it all week. It was a two-hour drive away with no traffic, but I was going to duck out early in case they were going to go to a strip club. Not only did I not want to go, but I wasn't sure if they wanted to go. Since he was marrying my wife's sister, I was technically a must-invite and therefore a snitch, so rather than cramp their style I opted out of knowing. I don't have anything against strip clubs, strippers or customers, I just don't like going there. When I was eighteen I went a couple times and at the time I was well over three hundred pounds and the attention I received was way too nice. It made me uncomfortable with the transactional nature of it and I've avoided them ever since. That said, I was looking forward to the rest of the day.

I met them all at a bar and they handed me a menu and watched as I read the whole thing. I ordered a beer a shot and a pizza and they cheered. If there was ever a crowd stoked to watch a dude eat pizza like he'd been doing exclusively for the past month, it was these guys. I saw them once or twice a year and we liked each other but didn't spend a lot of time on the phone or chatting over coffee, so they were super stoked to hear all about the diet. It was a month old and I had been talking about it every day for that entire month, so I was cool talking about it but internally I was hoping we wouldn't dwell on it for too much longer.

Until we didn't dwell on it for too much longer. Only one guy on this trip was single and you'd think if there was going to be a creeper at a party like this, it'd be the single guy, but it wasn't. He was just stoked to be there. He just finished a year of sobriety after kicking cancer for a second time and was just literally excited to be there. He was super casual about his triumph, too, in a way that made it even more impressive to hear about while we both lagged behind the group to avoid hearing the married father of three who was also a teacher describe his favorite part of every single female he saw.

The first couple times he said "goddamn! That ass!" I just replied with an "ew." unfortunately this seemed to have issued a challenge to him to find a part of a woman's body he could point out that would give me a boner to prove I wasn't gay or something, I don't know. I have never understood or appreciated when guys share things like this. After my disgust didn't work I tried going to the other extreme in hopes that maybe I could just get him to stand farther away from me. This was hard, but out creeping a creep is the most fun hobby I have. Nothing worked until he said something about "liking them young" and then I asked how old his daughter was and he finally got it.

No, he didn't get the fact that it's gross to comment on women's bodies like they were menu items, but he did excuse himself to the bar for a new beer and stood on the far end of the table when he got back, so I count that as a win. Bachelor parties aren't your last chance to cheat on your fiancé before she's your wife, and if they were, that rule would only apply to the bachelor, not the thirty-something married school teacher with three kids. Act like adults.

For dinner, I had oysters. Not oyster pizza, oyster oysters. I don't have strong opinions on pizza toppings with two exceptions: no ranch and never ranch. I don't like seafood, though, so the New Haven white pie doesn't sound appealing to me at all. Since that's the pizza from new haven, f you don't have it you don't get an opinion on the genre. One day I will have to choose to pretend to like it to fit in or be honest and be labeled a contrarian or a troll. In any case, on this night I had oysters and they were fine. I had been sobering up for a few hours and the plan was to bounce out after dinner and let these dudes rage with no snitch to ask weird questions about their daughters.

It was about eleven pm by the time I got back to my car. I intended to drive an hour north to my mother in law's house, sleep, then wake up the next morning and finish the drive home. Out of curiosity, I wanted to see how long the whole drive would take. I sat in my car and pulled up google maps on my phone, and as I typed in my home address I felt a sudden pressure on my car door. It wasn't a pressure like it had been hit, but like someone was leaning on it.

It felt like someone leaning on it because there was someone leaning on it. I could see the back of a head of long hair. My key was already in the ignition and my car was on but not running so I could roll down the window. I did. It was a woman.

"You ok?" I asked. Her shoulders tensed. She was cringing.

"Oh my god." she yelled. "Someone's in the car!" I looked past her and could see she was yelling at someone in the car parked next to mine -- a guy. He let out a mortified cackle. "I'm peeing!" she continued.

"Oh fuck, sorry." I rolled the window back up. My self-esteem was so low that I just apologized to a woman for catching her peeing on my car while I was sitting in it. Ordinarily I would've just spiraled, beating myself up for being weird, but I was powered by pizza. Through pizza anything is possible, and I needed to attack my weakness. I could still fix this! She was still peeing. I had to act fast and act big or I'd regret it for at least the entire drive home if not longer.

I rolled down the window again, and she immediately apologized. "I'm so sorry. There's no bathrooms and we sat in traffic for so long getting here and I was--"

"It's ok. I get it," I interrupted her. I'm a dude, we can pee wherever we want at any time for the most part, so it'd be wrong of me to judge someone else for doing the same thing just because they don't have the same gear as I do. Gear is code for penis. Even if she had a Shewee -- which is a thing they sell that combines a small cup and straw to mimic for a woman's anatomy how the penis moves urine out of a male's body, she wouldn't have years of practice with it to properly select a location to safely deploy it. The middle of a parking lot in downtown San Diego was a rookie choice, for sure.

Additionally, as what some people might consider an extreme endurance athlete with an autoimmune disease that directly affects my colon, I have been known, from time to time to need a bathroom in a hurry and it hasn't always ended well for me. If I were ever caught along some trail deep in the backcountry of the Santa Monica mountains, I would hope I would get the benefit of the doubt, so the benefit of the doubt is what I gave her. Napkins, actually, are what I gave. But they were an objective correlative for the benefit of the doubt I was giving, so it counts.

"Here's a couple napkins, if you need to wipe or whatever."

"Oh my god, thank you. You're very nice considering I'm peeing on your car." the guy in the car next to mine was still laughing, she was too. It was funny. Peeing on stuff is kind of funny.

It was late and though I looked forward to scoring some pizza at pizza port, near my mother in law's house halfway home, I truly just wanted to be home and sleep in my own bed and, yes, pee in my own toilet. Plus, had a kickball game the next day and needed to be well rested if I was going to win. I made the 2-and-a-half-hour drive like a breeze and was up early the next day, another preordained cheat day as it was a friend's birthday kickball party.

Playing kickball is super weird with seven stitches in your shin. But the weirdest part about the kickball party was how much I lost control over the diet. It was a potluck picnic style party at Griffith Park and we were going to play kickball on the grass. I brought pizza because I couldn't help myself. I was losing control. The experiment was bigger than me. The stupid rules we set up at the beginning did nothing about the extraordinary pressure to perform. On the other hand, I honestly still loved pizza so much that I would take any opportunity to eat it that I could get. I would dream about pizza. I would crave it. If I was eating pizza and smelled other pizza, I would get jealous.

I took the kickball too seriously and stopped having fun, so I had to stop playing. I brought running shoes just in case I needed to squeeze in an extra workout, but by the time I was done kickballing I just wanted to sit down and eat pizza, so that's what I did-- and when the party was over, I lobbied my wife hard to stop by a nearby Neapolitan pizza place that was my favorite in town. LA isn't as big as you'd think it'd be, but the travel time is insane. This pizza place is twelve miles from my house and if you went at the wrong time it could take up to ninety minutes. That's long enough to make even the best pizza too far away. That's long enough where running could be faster than driving. That's too long. So, when we're in the neighborhood I always try and stop in, regardless of what I had for lunch or dinner.

We did, and it was delicious. There's something special about Neapolitan pizza that sets it so far apart from most other thin crust styles. It's crunchy and chewy and airy and salty and the style is literally meant to be individual sized pies, so you don't even have to share. A good Neapolitan pie even has more whole looking ingredients: the pineapple is rough chopped, the pepperonis are hand torn, the sausage is all weird and scattered and the cheese is decidedly non-uniform. It just feels like you're back in the old country, sitting on your farm after a hard day's work picking grapes and olives and making wine and olive oil and then you just use whatever you got around to top off your daily pie. It's done before you even realize how tired and hungry you are, and then you drink some wine and go to sleep primed to do it all over again. If I had to choose a style of pizza, it would be "all you can eat," but if I had to choose a real style, I think it'd be Neapolitan.

After five weeks of The Great Pizza Experiment I was still down only eight pounds as working out was weird with a swollen, laced up shin. I didn't have any new powers to report but I was able to have lucid dreams, dreams in which you can do anything you want because you know it's a dream, in which I would eat copious amounts of pizza in hammocks and other comfortable pieces of furniture. Pizza was so deeply a part of my soul that I was in a dream in which I could fly, be a billionaire, do one-armed pull ups, or steal thoughts from the government but I was spending my lucid dreaming on pizza and loving it.

19. "POOR."

When I was a kid, we had a swimming pool in our backyard. I also had a ton of friends. One could say the two went hand in hand, but I was three when we moved into that house and we didn't leave for nine years. It's the longest I've ever lived in any place, so I literally have no idea what it would be like to grow up anywhere else or make friends without the benefit of being a kid with a pool. I was reasonably good at sports, hadn't yet become the three-hundred-pound monster of my late teens, and didn't have a problem making friends once I lived in a house without a pool, so I hesitate to say the pool was the only reason I had friends, but I know it could not have hurt.

Having a summer birthday and a pool made for some amazing parties, especially before I got all whaley and was too scared to take my shirt off in front of people. First, the obvious: a bunch of friends and sun and swimming is stereotypically awesome for a reason and if you haven't been alive long enough to learn to hate yourself and poison that well of fun, it lives up to the hype. Running, jumping, splashing, swimming, no school, a fuck ton of soda, ice cream cake, gifts, and most of all pizza. No shit I had a bunch of pizza at these summer parties. Pizza is an efficient way to feed a bunch of kids both in terms of calories, price, convenience and preference. Also, pizza is universally acceptable as a meal.

Since I had a summer birthday there wasn't any social pressure to invite any of the shitty kids from school. Elementary school is a social minefield in so many ways and inviting the right kids and skipping the wrong kids is crucial because if you get it half wrong or miss just one either way, everyone else is a witness and shit can get weird in a hurry. But when it was summer you were free. You could be the cool kid's token nerd friend or hang out with whomever you wanted without fear of judgment from the social elite and the elementary news cycle.

I didn't have those problems, specifically, because all my friends were dope. Even the one party I had where there was likely an attempted murder was still a blast for everyone involved, except the one dude that almost got drowned by the two others. The party that springs to mind is my eleventh. It would be my last birthday in the house with the pool, but I didn't know yet.

We came to California from New Jersey when I was three. I am from New Jersey. My wife always corrects me when I tell people I'm from back east. She hates it. She says, "you were born there you're not from there!" I was too young to have that place affect me at all, she says. I don't have any memories from living there, she says. Stop lying to people, you're from Claremont, Greg. I also sometimes claim I'm from New York City, which I can understand is a bit annoying because I claim it interchangeably with the New Jersey thing simply because if I remember neither, why not claim the one with more social credibility that's still technically true? I was born in Lenox Hill Hospital on Manhattan's Upper East Side, after all.

If I'm from Claremont it's this house I spent my childhood in that I'm from. It's the house that hosted a pizza eating contest on my eleventh birthday. We kept score by counting the crusts of our leftover slices. Looking back, I could have figured out that things weren't great financially for my parents, because for this party we had a bunch of pizza from a place called "The $2.99 Pizza Company."

The three-dollar pizzas came from the next town over, a decidedly lower income, neighborhood. It had a weird spice to it that I didn't like and could never explain, though now I could probably attribute it to a heavy hand with red pepper flakes in the sauce, or, god forbid, some jalapeno chopped up in there. There wasn't a good amount of cheese on it, either out I don't remember any of it being yellow or anything like that. You could tell by looking that it was cheap pizza.

We lived in a very nice white collar, middle class neighborhood. It wasn't upper middle class, but it wasn't a working-class neighborhood either. Our family did well for itself, but we weren't at the level of eating the bourgeois pizza chain pizza -- that was also the closest, every time we got pizza. That spot was for special occasions. Not fancy occasions, but also not Tuesday night and mom and dad are working late and didn't have time to plan a dinner. It was a family dinner place. We ate it off of glass plates. It was good pizza, but too expensive for a bunch of hyped up fifth graders to cram into their faces while dripping pool water all over the patio.

Typically, we'd bump down one to two tiers for parties. I don't want to name names or point fingers but we all know what pizza places are what tier in terms of quality. Every tier has its place in the grand scheme of things, sometimes you just want something quick and easy, other times you are ok spending a bit extra for a little bit better flavor in a place that'll have a nice area in which to wait, or some video games or a couple televisions. The three-dollar pizza company was not on this scale. I'm surprised there wasn't any bulletproof glass at the place, though I've had some delicious pizza that was passed through bulletproof glass. This three-dollar pizza was not that.

We kept score by counting crusts. As the entire party whittled down to contenders and finalists, we would lobby for others' leftover crusts, and so the contest transformed into a trophy crust contest. Years later I'd look back and compare the crusts piled on my and Jimmy's plates to the ears American GI's would collect during the Vietnam War for a body count, but that was in a poem I never published, and the metaphor was tenuous at best.

This wasn't killing some poor bastard who's just trying to defend his country and then dismembering his body, it was piling crusts on a plate. Eat a thousand pieces of pizza and pile up a thousand crusts and you will never come close to having a negative reaction akin to slicing an ear off a dead body. I reckon the worst part of saving the crust from a thousand slices of pizza would be not being able to eat the crust from a thousand slices of pizza!

I don't remember who won the contest, but it was my birthday, and this is my story, so I'll say I did. Despite that being my last birthday party in that house, despite that being the last summer I spent with a pool in my backyard, and even though we moved to the delivery area of the lowest tier pizza chain in town the next spring, that party and that pizza eating contest and those friends were perfect. Even if the mysteriously spicy pie ran out after our midnight swim with the pool lights off, around the same time we drained the last bit of dr. pepper and woke up my dad and pissed him off so bad he came out into the living room with his book and read to himself until we fell asleep it was an awesome party and an awesome house and you should've seen the pool.

THE GREAT PIZZA EXPERIMENT

20. "GUNPLAY."

Delivering pizzas for Firehouse Pizza in Riverside, California was one of the best jobs I have ever had in my life. It had everything I wanted: access to pizza, freedom, solitude, cash and interaction with a lot of people that I wouldn't have ever met were it not for the job. The complaints were normal enough. So and so isn't pulling their own weight. Customers are the actual worst. I hate mopping. The actual bad stuff, though, in life and in pizza delivery is so bad that you can't even complain about it.

The worst delivery of my life was to a little hotel near the airport. We never delivered to the hotel, not as a matter of policy but no guests there ever ordered. When I got there, I didn't know anything about which room was where and what was what. It wasn't that big of a hotel. I guess you'd call it a motel because it didn't have a lobby? I parked my car in the middle near the stairs and tried to suss out some kind of order of the rooms, so I could find the one on the ticket. It was upstairs, so I hit the stairs in the middle. I was a couple rooms away when the door flew open and an Indian man came running out yelling, "you kicked me, you kicked me!" and then there was an Indian woman in the parking lot yelling up to him, but I didn't hear what she was saying. The Indian man yelled back to the Indian woman in the parking lot and headed for the stairs at the other end of the building.

I kept approaching for some reason. I was one room down when a Latina woman left the open room, turned away and started down the same stairs as the Indian man who was now in the parking lot. A white dude came out of the room and he was yelling at the Indian guy who was still down in the parking lot yelling. That's when I saw a black pistol in his hand as he

125

watched the Latina woman get to the stairs. I froze for a second. He was my customer. I did not want to sell him this pizza. He was in the middle of some type of crazy motel fight and if I tried to sell this pizza to him I'd be involved in the crazy motel fight instead of just being around it. He held the gun so lightly and casually like it was a long neck beer and he was at a barbeque. He was not at a barbeque, though, he was in the early stages of a shootout and waiting for a pizza. A pizza I was holding in the big dumb insulated bag that is somehow the best way to keep pizza warm and probably is, but I worked in that pizza place over a year and never cleaned one ever.

I was on his gun side. He ordered the pizza forty-five minutes before I got there. If he was hungry when he called, he was hungrier now. If he saw me standing there, holding his pizza, who knows what he would do. He already had a gun out. For someone to pull a gun is crazy. This crazy would not be logically opposed, in my opinion, to sticking the gun they're already about to be in a ton of trouble for in the face of a pizza guy. I made minimum wage. The Latina woman he was watching made it to the stairs and the Indian man and woman - the motel manager and his wife were yelling about calling the police. I did what I do best: ran.

Running with a heat bag or whatever the technical name for that thing is, is hard but I managed to make it back to the stairwell and out of sight before the white dude saw me. Police sirens sounded and approached rapidly. If the white guy with the gun was following me, I was a dead person. The noose was tightening, and he had nothing to lose. Running down the stairs would make too much noise and then I would have to cross his field of fire to my car. The police cars skidded into the parking lot and there was a lot of commotion. I cowered in the corner of the stairwell and started eating his pizza. Thirty minutes later and with no shots fired he was under arrest and his pizza was all gone.

It was a ten-minute trip at most so when I got back to the shop an hour later everyone had a bunch of questions, most of which started angry but then calmed down a bit. Soon we were laughing about it. Not all of us laughed. Mostly just the owner who used to deliver pizzas told me about a couple times she was robbed back in the day. We joked about the guy in the

THE GREAT PIZZA EXPERIMENT

motel room next door and whether or not he might've wanted a pizza. I should've started knocking on doors after the cops left and seen if anyone wanted a pizza. I could've made a sale despite the rough circumstances, she laughed. I countered and unveiled a new rule: if I see a gun, whatever I'm delivering belongs to me. It could be my last meal after all.

I was joking but the truth is I was very lucky to only have seen one gun in the fifteen months I spent delivering pizzas. I was doubly lucky that I only saw the side of the gun. Some people aren't so lucky. In fourth grade, I was shopping at a local supermarket with my parents. We were back by the butcher when we heard a bunch of yelling. Then a couple quick pops and flashes and more yelling. We hid behind an end cap until my dad said it was safe. The store was robbed, and a woman was shot. When it was safe we just continued shopping, checked out and went home.

We wouldn't get the full story until the next day in the paper. The store was robbed at gunpoint by two men. As they were running to their car they shot a woman in the parking lot. The woman was walking into the store from her pizza shop across the parking lot. She was trying to trade some money for quarters and they shot her, and they got away. She survived and would make a full recovery. She was very lucky. A different kind of luck than mine.

I never knew why they would just shoot a random woman while escaping. How did they know she had a bunch of money? I was suspicious. My mom was a cog on the small-town rumor mill and in that position, she caught a lot of gossip. A lot of unverifiable gossip. Like the fact that the manager of that Straw Hat Pizza wasn't just a manager of a Straw Hat Pizza. She was an undercover cop trying to infiltrate some type of drug trade. In her cover job as pizza restaurateur she came across the robbers, broke cover and pulled her gun and that's when the shot her and took all her shit.

I have not been able to find a single source to corroborate that version of events. This fact would be suspicious if I could find one single source to corroborate that the store I was in when it was robbed, and a woman was shot was robbed and a woman was shot. There is no record of any of what happened. There is no official account. There may be microfiche in some dusty library basement somewhere that has so far escaped digitization, I don't know. I'm not suggesting a conspiracy theory here. I'm being very clear about my experience, the unsubstantiated rumors I heard and a very small amount of research I've conducted. The woman never returned to work at the pizza place and it changed ownership soon after the robbery. This is consistent with an owner who took a bullet in the line of duty. Whether she ate everything in the store before quitting as I would have or not, though, remains unclear.

21. "DESSERT."

After five full weeks of The Great Pizza Experiment I was down a total of eight pounds and could control my own dreams. My life was going great. I don't know if it was just the pizza or a concert of everything going amazingly and nothing going poorly that made me feel like I was soaring, and it showed. My skin glowed like I was pregnant, and I smiled an uncomfortable proportion of the time. I had nothing to fear and no worries. More money would have been cool, but more money always makes things a little better so that doesn't count.

It was time to get my stitches out and I couldn't wait to get back out on the road and not have that weird feeling in my leg. The only thing keeping me down was not being able to move freely. The extraction was uneventful, and you know I had pizza afterwards to celebrate. I went back to work and finished all my assignments for the day, had another slice and then stared out the window and drifted off into thought.

I only ate cheese pizza until I was sixteen. It's not all I ate, but it was the only type of pizza I ate. It was a simple life and very tasty. Not a wide spectrum but that was my palate and it was all I knew and all I liked. I was living my truth and for me at the time that was all I liked. When people didn't order cheese pizza, it was more than an inconvenience for me, it was an attack on my way of life.

"Just peel it off," said every single grown up person ever, like they had never seen pepperoni in their entire lives. When you cook pepperoni the fat renders and mixes into the cheese. This is no secret. That is straight up science, but adults would just lie to me and tell me it was fine when I

129

knew it wasn't. Turning pepperoni pizza into cheese pizza by pulling the pepperonis off is like trying to un-chew food, it doesn't work! I'm surprised this pepperoni conspiracy didn't scar me for life with regards to trusting authority, to be quite honest. It did take the edge off when I figured out that all grownups lie all the time, though, which was nice.

Worse than the pepperoni conspiracy was a stray olive. Olives are the worst. If you combined the worst part of salt with the platonic ideal of bitterness and hide it in a package with five-star yelp reviews and weird textures and then you add a fucking pit that nobody ever complains about or seems to notice? Give me a fucking break. Olives? You're all fucking liars. I've had one olive in my life that I would consider half as good as all you sociopaths claim they are and it was directly from a friend's olive grove in Syria. Fuck all other olives especially hitchhiker olives that show up on otherwise oliveless pizzas. Wash your fucking pizza cutters you goddamn scuzzbuckets.

Growing up, every Friday was the best because: no school for two days and Friday nights were pizza nights. This Friday, the sixth Friday of The Great Pizza Experiment, was more special than those Fridays as a kid though. It was more special than those Fridays as a kid because I had had nothing but pizza for almost forty days leading up to it and I was supposed to have pizza that day. It was like a month with three paydays or finding twenty dollars in an old jacket and then finding fifty dollars in the other pocket every day for almost forty days and then waking up in the morning and knowing you were going to find that money in the jacket again. It was an amazing Friday.

It was an amazing day, except for one small detail: it was free pizookie day. The pizookie is BJ's Pizza's version of a desert pizza. It has a scoop of ice-cream on top and it comes out in a still hot skillet, so you have no choice but to eat it quickly before the ice cream turns to cream cream. This is the perfect dessert: flavor, texture, wildly different temperatures and best of all a ticking clock so nobody could judge you for eating too fast because it's melting! Unfortunately for The Great Pizza Experiment pizookies are cookies. This is the only bad thing about pizookies. It's cookie dough, there's no sauce, no toppings just fillings or different types of cookie dough. It was clear to me. It was so clear I didn't even need to ask. What standards did I use to determine this fact? My eyes. I looked with my eyes and had I not the benefit of the menu and the advertising and branding I would say "wow that is a big cookie," not "wait. Is that a pizza or a cookie or both?"

In the fifteen hours I was awake on free pizookie day I was forced to explain that a pizookie was not a pizza no less than one hundred times. I'm still grumpy about it because the only thing worse than not being able to eat a giant cookie topped with ice cream for free, is having to explain to a hundred smiling faces who just wanted a shred of involvement in the greatest experiment of all time that they were wrong about what constitutes a pizza, rude for rubbing it in my face that I couldn't eat it, and completely unoriginal because literally everyone else asked me the same dumb question. I probably kept my cool about it, though, because I took the edge off with a milkshake at lunch.

I earned that milkshake. I had a job interview at lunch time and no private area to take the call, so I took it in my car. It was October in southern California and not a cold one. I was parked in the sun, but my back windows are tinted so I figured it'd be ok. It was not ok. It was so hot in the car that by the end of the call when I was loopy and comparing on air promotions - the field in which I am employed, to poetry - the field in which I took my Bachelor of Arts, which is the Schrödinger's cat of insight freshman year of college type shit). I had sweat through two shirts and my underwear was soaked so thoroughly that it looked like I put my pants on over a wet swimsuit. It was so bad that when I got back to work people kept asking if I was ok. How anyone leaves their animals in hot cars is beyond me. I wonder if I blacked out in the heat and said a bunch of crazy shit or if the "promos are the poetry of entertainment," was enough for the hard pass, but either way I did not get the job.

The weekend brought me to a dodger game. The dodgers are my favorite sports team. The dodgers are objectively the best team in the history of sports, so it's no wonder that going to their games makes me very happy. They inspired me as a kid to play and practice and had I not quit playing baseball to audition for an improv troupe (fuck.) I could've been on the dodgers, probably. The dodgers also got me a job. I commented on a dodger's bobblehead doll in the hiring manager's office and then we swapped memories for the entire interview and the offer came the next week and the job was awesome.

The dodgers just needed to cleave their way into my experiment to solidify their position as best thing of all time. And cleave their way in they did. I was on a strict pizza only diet - if you recall, but I was in the house of the best hotdog on earth: the eponymous dodger dog. I was emotionally weak after the free pizookie Friday and I could tell I was vulnerable. I needed to fill up on pizza fast to avoid the poor choices that result from cravings and lowered inhibitions from baseball game beer.

Los Angeles baseball stadium pizza is about as unappealing as it sounds, but the dodgers have a secret weapon: Uncle Tommy. Tommy LaSorda is the quintessential dodger - a scrappy but successful transplant from Brooklyn who is now beloved in his adopted hometown. He is referred to as Uncle Tommy in my and many other households in Los Angeles and across the nation. He's such an important guy I keep a picture of him on my phone. It's a picture of him and my mom, but I have a lot of better pictures of her on my phone, this one I have because of Tommy.

He's of Italian descent, so when they updated the in-stadium dining options, they gave him his own joint. Lasorda's Trattoria was out in the right field pavilion and did sausage and peppers, pizza, pasta, Peroni, and probably garlic fries. It was on the complete other side of the stadium from where I was sitting but I would not abide by domino's pizza, which is the only other choice in the park. I walked past twenty places to buy dodger dogs on the way over there. I was struggling. I got in line and before I had a chance to fully digest the menu it was my turn.

An angel sang. The crowd erupted in pure joy. The world went white and my vision narrowed to a single glorious sight. My true love. Inside the plastic display case on the counter was a slice of cheese, a slice of pepperoni and a pizza pretzel - which is just a dumb pretzel, let's not get into it. Underneath all of those things was another slice of cheese, but the crust was elevated. The tag on the case said, "Dodger Dog Stuffed Crust Pizza." It is exactly what it sounds like: a piece of pizza with the world's most famous hotdog stuffed into the crust. I don't know if I ordered two of them or just rapped the glass and grunted but I ate them before I realized what happened and brought a third back to the seats. My friends applauded the match made in heaven. Real respects real and they saw the truth that day and they clapped.

Looking back, I could've just put a hotdog on top of the pizza, but I literally just thought of that now, a full three years after the day of record. I missed out on a lot of cravings not just dropping them onto a pizza and calling them toppings. It's not like I had any qualms about it, either, it's what did for the first meal of the dang diet. That's how glorious the dodger dog is, it had me shook. Even though I was programmed to eat pizza, I was drawn to it. And relieved, to be honest, that it was combined with pizza for me because I definitely wouldn't have thought about it until much too late.

I was also a bit behind the curve as far as cognition as I was drinking beer at an incredible rate, which doesn't lend itself well to problem solving. Coincidentally it also inhibits weight loss. On the Monday following the sixth week of The Great Pizza Experiment I had, again, no change in weight from week to week due to that proper day-drinking session that turned into a bit of an all-nighter. Looking back, I'm lucky I didn't gain weight week to week, but such is the miracle of an all pizza diet: there's no way to gain weight no matter how hard you try. That is a lie. You need to work your ass off if you're going to try this.

22. "THE PIZZA EXPERIENCE."

My wife was a suit at an advertising agency. It was stressful. She ended up leaving and she was relieved beyond measure. She took a week in Bali to detoxify her soul because she's fancy, and that was the minimum effective dose. When she came back she knew she made the right choice, but also had a restlessness in her that is one of my favorite things about her. She has this energy - when she's not napping, that is urgent and endearing. She's also brilliant and fun. This isn't about why I love my wife, this is about her business.

She was the person best able to testify to the true power of pizza, for it was pizza that broke her from her ill-conceived ideas about the superiority of sandwiches. She was also deep into Pinterest and aesthetics, for better or for worse. Better because wherever we go and whatever we do, we come back with great pictures to remember the moment. Worse because each one of those pictures detracts from each moment, especially after the ninth take!

Near the end of The Great Pizza Experiment, when I was injured, started reminiscing about pizza moments of my life. When The Great Pizza Experiment was over I was thinking about ways to go back in time and relive my best life which, as I've already discussed at length, was the life of a man who ate nothing but pizza. Since I had a degree in creative writing, had always threatened to write a book, had several awards for writing, and was in fact a professional writer, naturally I thought of writing a fictionalized version as a feature film. Then I remembered that I was not very good at writing feature films -- at least according to most of my screenwriting instructors in undergrad as well as grad school. The next best idea was a television pilot, but it was a limited series at best. I dipped into the memory bank and withdrew my memories from the year and change that I spent washing dishes and delivering pizzas and everything else at a pizza place in college for my inspiration before realizing that nobody buys tv pilots from people who've never sold a tv pilots. A play would be boring or whatever. I actually don't know as I've seen a frighteningly few number of plays in my life.

I was admittedly naive about the world of publishing, so I began writing this book, not to finish writing a book and get it published, but because that's what I learned in college: write, rewrite, rewrite, rewrite, rewrite, gap, make a living. The gap part was considered too gauche a topic for the hallowed writing workshop.

I worked almost exclusively during episodes of the bachelor and the bachelorette. When I started writing the book, I would bring my laptop to another room and write alone, but I actually like my wife and being away from her to slave away at work was more unbearable than working through the show I used to dismiss as trash. After a while I would actually learn to love the show enough to risk my kidneys on it -- remember rhabdo? I finished the first draft while my wife was in Bali, and this was the big news when she got back.

Roughly two weeks later, during the bachelor of course, she paused the show and said, "I have a thought..." My wife keeps things interesting. For example, when I'm seconds away from falling asleep after we've said good night, I might get a question that begins "if you were a squirrel...." so I naturally figured it was a squirrel kind of question. She continued, "so this book you're writing, right now you'll probably just sell a few online to family and friends, but what if we sold it in the gift shop of pizza pop-up museum? I'm gonna do that!" And at that moment, The Pizza Experience pop-up museum was born.

I just figured, yeah yeah ok sure. We all have lofty dreams. I'm writing a book I don't know what I'm going to do with and she can create a museum on the side. We'll never put a deadline on either and that will be that. A week later, she trapped me with a presentation and excel sheet of pizzas and experiential art and market research when I was stretched out on the couch after a pair of back to back long runs that turned me into a blob, half drunk and unable to escape. She loves to trap me on Friday nights to look at excel sheets. After I saw her pitch, I was convinced. She hired me as creative consultant. My salary was beer and I spent the next few weekends locked in either a beer hall or our kitchen, being force fed beers and riffing ideas. I say riffing because even though I was being paid with beer for my ideas, the concepts we arrived at were greater than the sum of our individual ideas. She brought in a friend who was in the experiential marketing field, and then the ideas took off.

She would pitch me plans and they were huge in scope, insurmountable in difficulty, and crazy in inception. Most of these conversations would involve a lot of PowerPoint presentations and every slide me saying something like, "what? That's crazy!" or, "you can do that?" Because most of it was super logical but I had always taken things like this for granted. She'd say things like "I'm going to rent a space," and I was blown away. I don't know why. It makes sense that every business has a space that they need to rent, but it was outside the scope of my needs and so I had honestly never considered it.

I was mired in the cant's and the how's, but she was cold calling suits and setting up sponsorships. She was interviewing fabricators, setting up payroll, meeting with commercial real estate brokers, and doing everything that's ever been done to set up a company. I went to work every day and would get briefed on the day's progress. It was all amazing. This was stuff that grown ass adults would do and she was just doing it. I've worked at one company since college. I've had three different jobs but if i went my way I would've just been promoted instead of moving jobs. I'll spare you the millennials-get-a-bad-rap-from-baby-boomers-for- being itinerant-and-poor-but-the-world-is-different-for-us-and-it's-the-boomers'-

ault rant. Mostly because I'm too lazy to type it out. My point is, I've done ne grown up thing in my life, and I've just been riding that wave ever since.

Chasing your dreams is fucking terrifying and seeing my wife face hat fear every day with poise, courage and strength was uplifting as all hell. he literally lifted me up, sometimes tugging me along by my earlobe or ollar or whatever metaphor best fits her checking monthly, then weekly, hen daily about the progress on my book, this book, so she could sell it in he gift shop. Eventually it stopped being "how's your book?" and started eing "you have twenty weeks until your book is finished, printed and in my ift shop. If it is not done and done well, you will be embarrassed."

Big problem. That meant I'd have to finish the book and sell it. To inish the book, I would have to work hard and then let people read it. etting people read it would mean friends and family, who figure very eavily into the work would read it. With my book in their hands, I would ave nowhere to hide. That's the thing about books. Real books. If I wrote iction I wouldn't give a shit like my screenplays and pilots as the only risk howing those is that people could think I'm a bad writer, which I know I am ot. Showing my memoir to people, even if it's just the pizza parts, might nake them think I'm a bad person, which I only think I am not. So here is my nner self, pepperonis and stray olives and all. If you don't like it, blame my vife.

23. "CATHARSIS."

I had been eating nothing but pizza for the past six weeks and over that amount of time I had lost eight pounds. I had been lauded, tested, and congratulated and was very much enjoying my victory lap. I was traveling to New Orleans at the end of the seventh week. I knew The Great Pizza Experiment was going to come to an end, so for the five days of this week I chose to savor every moment of being allowed to eat the greatest food on earth for every meal not only without judgement but to voracious crowd approval.

A victory lap is that moment after the race where you drape yourself in your country's flag and jog around the stadium saying hi to everyone and thanking them for their support, weeping and waving at the admiring masses in the stands and watching on tv at home. Mine was the same, but from my favorite pizza places in town, the ones that held my hand and led me through the promised land. My first stop on the Gregory Boytos pizza tour was 800 degrees pizza. It was as empty as it always was and as I came in they greeted me like they always did when the door opened. But then one of them said "oh hey Greg. Getting the Instagram special again today?" I shed a single tear. To be called out by name and have a usual order is a monument to consistency, dedication, and sacrifice, and to achieve that on my own for the first time in my life on the corner of sunset and vine - one of the busiest most crowded street corners in one of the most crowded cities on earth, made it more than special. I was a pizza legend.

The next stop was a very popular, trendy place very close to work. i was one of those chef-made pizza places that uses inventive toppings and also does espresso, baked goods and pastries. It's one of those places that ends up on a blog, so you say you'll try it and then you do, and you wait in line and pay a little bit more than you normally would, and it's fine but ordinarily you'd just skip it. This was that place but six months later when the business volume matched the quality of the product. It was a good pizza, so the place was far from empty and at lunch and dinner times I'd have to squeeze into the bar to avoid waiting for a table.

I had a butternut squash pizza. It was a handsome pie with a lot of colors and great burn marks. They cut it into tiny square pieces and it was just begging to be photographed. I pulled out my phone and stopped in my tracks. I had an out of body experience and could see myself from above. I saw a thirty-year-old man, overweight, balding, wearing a cat shirt, sitting alone in front of a pizza big enough for two people at a bar at lunch in the middle of the week. It was a sad sight.

There was a group of young people sitting down the bar a little bit loudly talking shit about everything, which made it worse. This would be the exact group of people to call out an old person for trying to do young people shit in public, like rollerblading or skateboarding or food photography. They could've been goddamn influencers and their cruel snipe about the sad old drunk taking pictures of his food could've made me a meme before I got back to the office couch for my post-lunch nap. They say discretion is the better part of valor, and so instead of risking taking the picture and being exposed as an old fraud, I put my phone back in my pocket and finished my pizza. Later, I found a picture of that restaurant's butternut squash pizza on Google and posted it which was, for me, preferable to risking ridicule at the hands of millennials and I regret nothing.

I had a dentist appointment the next day. I schedule my dentist appointments for lunchtime because my dentist is very near my office. My dentist is cool as fuck. He's the only dentist I've ever had in my entire life that isn't stingy with Mr. Thirsty (the vacuum straw they use to suck the spit out of your mouth). I'm hella juicy mouthed in general so there's a lot of spit, but I also have some weird post nasal drip that bothers me if I can't swallow it. The Mr. Thirsty thing is huge for my comfort. It's a courtesy that I very much appreciate, so I try and return the same level of courtesy by not showing up to breathe on him with an empty stomach because nothing smells worse than empty stomach breath.

I usually get a chicken salad across the street. It's one of my favorite salads in town. That was not available to me as I was on an all pizza diet, so had to improvise. There was a local pizza chain right next door to the dentist, but it wasn't anything to write home about. It's expensive, the dough is too dense and dry, and the toppings aren't the best. Sometimes the crust is like half of the pizza, which would be fine, but the crust is like a thick, rubbery cracker. Their beer list was ok, though, so I had been there a few times before.

I was feeling adventurous, so I picked a random pie and went with it. The only thing was I didn't know what one of the words were. I had never seen it before and it was the letterhead topping of the pie I had chosen, Nduja. It was my turn to order and I stepped up to the register. I tried to hooked on phonics it and make the N silent while also hitting the J pretty hard. While I did this, I held up the menu and pointed to the pie I wanted to order so the cashier would know I didn't know how to pronounce it.

Apparently, I pronounced it quite wrong because his eyes shot wide and he started laughing out loud. He was so aggressively laughing about my flub that he didn't even do that thing where you cover your mouth or turn your head so the people you're laughing at can't see you laughing. My shoulders dropped, and he realized he was laughing at me and regained control. He apologized and corrected me. Apparently, you pronounce the N like you're about to say "No," very nicely, and then the J is soft. It sounds like something Dirty Harry would growl at a criminal, and apparently, it's just a spicier version of soppressata and a bit thicker.

I ate it because I had no other options, but it tasted like bullying and pepper and the pineapple wasn't sweet enough to make up for it. Too much crust, too, if we're being honest. Spent the next hour on my back breathing pepper cured pork onto my dentist, a hundred percent sure he would subtweet it later to all his dentist friends about how the old balding guy with the cat shirt had Nduja breath and was also fat. That was the last time I went to that pizza shop. Mostly because there's better non-pizza options around and I'm no longer on an all pizza diet but getting laughed at that hard is enough for me to boycott. I've boycotted for less.

I didn't wear jeans from 1993 until 2009 because I was upset that it was socially acceptable for jeans to have holes, but not sweatpants. Pockets on jeans are also terrible. They're cut too tight for egress, ingress or regress while standing and are positively sealed while sitting. The pockets also are on the front of your legs instead of the side, so you can break whatever's in there if you sit down too quickly without properly aligning it. This was an official boycott and it only ended because my wife wanted to see me in jeans.

In 2001, I smoked a bunch of pot with my friends and went to a fast food restaurant which shall remain nameless. It was named after a girl though and they have square burgers which are an abomination and a crime against nature. I ordered chicken nuggets or whatever the fuck those dumbshits call them, and small fries. When the food came out there was no sauce. I like BBQ sauce with my nugs because as we've established I have excellent taste and the best judgement with regards to food. I asked for BBQ sauce and they said extra sauce was twenty-five cents. That's a quarter. That is not a lot of money. BBQ sauce, however is not on the menu, therefore I could not independently verify that the sauce was this much money, plus, it wasn't extra, it was just one.

"Those don't come with sauce. It's twenty-five cents." The way she said it made me one hundred percent sure that this was non-negotiable. Also, I was pretty stoned, so I slid a quarter across the counter and got my sauce. I went back to the table and ate. The BBQ sauce was well worth the quarter. It tasted so good. I went to grab a handful of fries to temper the sweetness of the BBQ sauce with some saltiness. The first handful of fries were fucking delicious. Perfect. I was high though, so they obviously tasted like they were frozen.

Wait, what? Pot doesn't make stuff taste cold. I took another bite. Straight up ice. Frozen cooked potatoes. Gross. I brought the fries back to my friend behind the counter. She saw me standing there but didn't move an inch until I spoke up.

"Excuse me, these fries are frozen." I slid the fries across the counter to her.

"OK," she said. That was it. She went back to doing nothing and waiting for me to speak.

"I can't eat them."

"OK," she said and threw them in the trash. Then we played chicken. I don't know how long I stood there while I waited for a resolution, but it never came.

"Fuck this!" I said, probably not very loud because: coward, and walked outside and sat on the curb near my friends' car while they finished their food. I was insulted, horrified and confused. I vowed to never return to that place and have stayed so true to that vow that I won't even ride in a car through their drive through on road trips when I'm outvoted by shitty friends. Which is all to say, I'll never go back to that mean pizza place Nduja know what I mean?

That night was a special night. Usually I would train after work, have a smoothie and go to sleep but this night there was a party. My friend Erik was appearing on Jeopardy. He was having a viewing party at a bar near UCLA that did a pretty decent bar pie. I was itching for anything to erase the pain of the afternoon savagery I experienced so I was more than excited to attend. It was relatively uneventful as my friend Erik lost to that weird Jeopardy champion, which is about as specific I can get and unfortunately covers the bulk of the multiday champions in recent memory. He kept up through single Jeopardy, but the defending champion's use of game theory allowed him to pull away from Erik and the other contestant and secure yet more money for his final pot.

The episode was shot months before. A lot of game shows are shot in advance, google it. I don't work on jeopardy or for a company that is affiliated with the production or distribution of jeopardy as far as I know. The bet I had with my wife and the experiment I continued after the quick victory were made independent of everything Alex Trebek related. As far as I'm concerned, my life and Jeopardy are on opposite ends of the universe, yet there on that episode on that night during the seventh and final week of The Great Pizza Experiment, was an entire category dedicated to pizza. I went five for five, of course, and to be sure there was no category related in any way to sandwiches.

The last day of The Great Pizza Experiment was Friday as I was heading to New Orleans with my wife to meet up with some college friends. I was very much looking forward to it as I was obsessed with New Orleans as a kid up to and including applying to Tulane University as a high school senior, before withdrawing my application after 9/11 because I didn't want to be far from home. I woke up that day full of gratitude in a way I only could have felt after forty-four days eating only pizza. I've done some amazing stuff in my life but waking up that morning was the most whole I had ever felt up until that point in my life and I have not felt that way since.

I was floating through life. I weighed myself like I had every day of The Great Pizza Experiment and discovered I was only down nine pounds total. This was suboptimal. Here I was trying to make a point about popular diets and diet fads by losing weight despite eating a taboo food and I had a measly single digit loss. Sure, I had lost two weeks of training due to a freak accident, but diet books don't care about excuses. They care about referring to cherry picked studies out of context that nobody will ever read and heaps of testimonials. They are the original clickbait. I had to juke the stats a little bit the same way every other diet book excludes studies that don't suit its purpose, ignore obvious confirmation bias, or complain about how difficult it is to perform controlled studies on diets because of the money and the oversight required to make sure people follow the study and the government is involved somehow and big pharma too, and some different food lobbies are also interfering but trust them, their dang diet works!

The Great Pizza Experiment may have been a joke, but it could not be a lie. It never occurred to me that I could just lie about the amount of weight I lost until I began writing this book. You read that right. I was so infused with the beauty of pizza that the darkness of lies never shone on my heart. I did need results, however, so I went out for a ten-kilometer run and when I got back I was four pounds lighter, making the final weight loss thirteen pounds. This was acceptable. This was almost two pounds per week which is a good number!

The final stats of The Great Pizza Experiment were remarkable. The experiment lasted forty-five days. The total weight lost was thirteen pounds. I had run a total of forty miles. I had burned a total of eight thousand and five hundred calories doing high intensity interval training workouts in my garage. I had swum a total of eight miles. I had eaten a grand total of thirty one pizzas which translates to at least two hundred and forty-eight slices if we're talking about New York style and almost five hundred if one were dealing in classic American style pizzas. The reality is somewhere in between as I didn't specify total number of slices consumed, only total number of pies.

The Great Pizza Experiment was over with the final weigh in, and had to grab some lunch before we hopped on a plane to The Big Easy. I was excited to finally be unchained from The Great Pizza Experiment and be allowed to eat whatever I wanted. I went to Little Caesars and got a five dollar pizza and for the first time in a month and a half, I got a side of crazy bread too. I ate the whole bag of crazy bread while the pizza was cooking and it was so good I almost wept. Infused with the same kind of crazy that makes the crazy bread so fantastic, I made an honest effort to buy a six foot by eight foot poster of crazy bread from the store, but the lady wasn't able to sell it to me and the manager wasn't there and I didn't want to wait for them to come back because halfway through my conversation I lost interest in owning the poster so I just left, ate my pizza and went to the airport.

That night in New Orleans, after drinking the dumbest tourist drink we could find and just about anything else we came across, me and my wife and our crew of college friends raged through the French Quarter the way only thirty-year old married couples can. We fit right in, unfortunately but we weren't trying to not be tourists so it's fine. We had beignets, and cafe au lait and we talked about pizza and sandwiches. It was four AM before any of us even thought about wrapping it up for the night, but as soon as someone said it, the flood gates opened, and everyone was in vehement agreement. We all started the long walk back to our hotel together, but to the group's amazement, I had to duck into an all-night pizza shop for a slice to head off the next morning's hangover.

ABOUT THE AUTHOR

Gregory Boytos is the co-creator of The Pizza Experience – a multisensory pizza pop-up (www.the-pizza-experience.com), an award winning screenwriter, poet, producer, comedic improvisor and ultra-endurance athlete. He can be found at www.gregoryboytos.com on Instagram as @thepizzathlete and at The Improv Space in the world famous Westwood neighborhood of Los Angeles. He is a devout Los Angeles Dodgers and New York Giants fan and an outspoken cat person.

33925601R00084

Made in the USA
Middletown, DE
20 January 2019